TRIALS OF A NURSING STUDENT

Tips to Successfully Sail Through Nursing School and Beyond

●━━━━━━━━●

Wynisha Alcorn MSN, RN

Library of Congress Cataloging-in-Publication Data

Library of Congress Control Number:2019908554

Wynisha Alcorn MSN, RN
TRIALS OF A NURSING STUDENT: Tips to Successfully Sail Through Nursing School and Beyond
Published by: Wynisha Alcorn:
PO Box 1965 League City, TX 77574

ISBN: 9781075802669

Disclaimer
All contents of this book are given for informational and educational purposes only. The author is not in any way accountable for any results or outcomes that emanate from using this material. Constructive attempts have been made to provide information that is both accurate and effective, but the author is not bound for the accuracy or use/misuse of this information.

Table of Contents

Acknowledgements vii
Introduction: How to Use This Book................................... 1

Chapter One: Set Yourself Up to Succeed............................... 5

7 Tips to Prepare Your Life for Nursing School
Essential Nursing Supplies Shopping List
Essentials Shopping List
Nice-to-Haves List
Nursing School Preparation Checklist
Essential Nursing Supplies Checklist

Chapter Two: What to Expect in Nursing School: Five Things the Brochure Doesn't Mention... 23
1. Nursing school burnout is normal and preventable
2. It will cost you more than you expect
3. You will want to quit
4. Choose your friends wisely
5. You will need to get used to foul smells...quickly
Chapter Summary and Putting it into Action

Chapter Three: A Day in the Life of a Successful Nursing Student and How to Structure Your Day................................. 34
A Day in the Life of a Successful Nursing Student
How to Balance Nursing School with Life
Create Your Quiet Space
Remember You Are Doing It for Them
Plan to Make Time for Relationships
Make Your Own Schedule for Success in Four Easy Steps
Step #1 Start with your priorities in mind
Step #2 Choose your method of schedule keeping
Step #3 Build your master schedule
Step #4 Plan to plan

How to Find Time to Study When You're a Parent
Chapter Summary and Putting it into Action

Chapter Four: How to Dominate Stress and Anxiety..........46
Stress Throws You Off Your Game
The What, How, and Why of Stress?
Dominating Stress
Beat Test Anxiety
Chapter Summary and Putting it Into Action

Chapter Five: How to Maximize Your Study Time and Ace Your Exams.. 58
Pomodoro Technique
Note taking Methods and Tips
Take Notes on Lecture Slides
Use Technology
The Old-Fashioned Way
Four Note taking Tips
Know Your Learning Style and Use It
The Visual Learner
The Auditory Learner
The Kinesthetic Learner
Form a Study Group
Tips on How to Have a Successful Study Group
Use Social Media to Excel in Your Classes
Create Your Own Study Guides
More Tips to Avoid Distractions
Tutor Assistance
Discipline and Train Your Mind
Tips to Improve Your Memory and Brain Function
Chapter Summary and Putting it into Action

Chapter Six: Simple Keys to Success................................ 82
Set goals and read them daily
Treat teachers as coaches
Start a study group with the smartest students in your class
Take advantage of learning centers
Immerse yourself in your craft

Prioritize self-care
Chapter Summary and Putting it into Action

Chapter Seven: Clinical Do's and Don'ts............................. 88
Preparing for Clinicals as a Nursing Student
Clinical Do's and Don'ts for Success
A Note About Nursing Diagnosis
Chapter Summary and Putting it into Action

**Chapter Eight: How to Stick it Out When Nursing
School Gets Hard**.. 96
Dealing with Instructor Problems
How to Make Your Toughest Teacher Your Biggest Ally
Recognizing Intimidators at Work
Bullies
Racial and Gender Discriminators
Gender Bias and Discrimination
Dealing with Racism
Tips to Deal with Bullying and Discrimination in the
Workplace or School
Chapter Summary and Putting it into Action

**Chapter Nine: Everything You Need to Know About NCLEX
The NCLEX Breakdown**.. 110
How to Register for the NCLEX
What to Expect on the NCLEX
Tips to Prepare for the NCLEX Exam
What to Do if You Fail the First Time
Chapter Summary and Putting it into Action

**Chapter Ten: A Few More Quick Tips to Enjoy
Nursing School**.. 120
Tip #1 Stay Organized to Avoid Stress
Tip #2 Reward Yourself for Small Milestones
Tip #3 Make Time for Fun Weekly
Tip #4 Eat and Sleep

Tip #5 Be Mindful of the Moment
Tip #6 Think of College as Preparation for Your Dream Job
Chapter Summary

Chapter Eleven: Beyond Nursing School............................ 127
8 Surprising Things About Being a Nurse
Tips to Find Your Dream Nursing Job
Begin with a Clear Vision
Obtain References
Put Together a Strong Cover Letter and Resume
Tap into Your Network First
Utilize Social Media in Your Job Search
Search Job Listings Wisely
Build Experience You Need
Chapter Summary and Putting it into Action

Resources for Your Journey...137
Books and Audiobooks
General Nursing Books
Exam Preparation
Study Skills and Learning Styles
Nursing Specialties
Apps for Your Smartphone or Tablet
Blogs and Websites to Follow
General Nursing Blogs and Websites
Nursing Jobs
Podcasts
YouTube channels
Facebook groups
Miscellaneous Nursing Supplies

About the Author.. 151
Other Resources by Wynisha Alcorn MSN, RN.................. 152

Acknowledgements

First and foremost, I would like to thank God for giving me this opportunity to share my knowledge and experience to give hope to others in spite of life's circumstances.

I would like to acknowledge my amazing husband and best friend David for always loving and supporting me.

Thank you to my mother Angela (who is also a nurse) for being a mentor to me and for giving me life.

Thank you to my father Willie and stepmother Tanya for always being available and loving my children with ALL your hearts.

I'm grateful for family, for standing by my side when my life was in jeopardy following my stroke. I wouldn't be where I am today without your unconditional love and support.

Thank you to my grandmother Linda (who is also a retired nurse) for caring for my oldest son while I was in the hospital. You taught me how to love.

Thank you to my grandmother Lillie for taking care of my brother and me so my mother could attend nursing school.

I want to thank my brother Willie for helping with the care of my children while I healed.

To my children Pershaun, Ki'erra, David, and Dalyn, thank you for giving me the strength and motivation to keep going.

I would like to acknowledge all of my wonderful colleagues over the years. You are an inspiration to me and future generations of nurses.

Last, but certainly not the least, thank you to all of my nursing instructors for instilling in me the knowledge I have today. This book would not be possible without your guidance and encouragement. I'm sure I would have gotten my Nursing degree through traditional learning, but I will not be a N.U.R.S.E. (Nurturing, Understanding, Reliable, Selfless, Extraordinary) had it not been tough love shared equally amongst the class. Whether it was to get me excited, calm me down, or humble me, I always walked away from the conversation a better professional.

Introduction: How to Use This Book

Congratulations! You've decided to become a nurse, so you signed up for nursing school. This is an exciting time. You are preparing for a career that will completely change your life. You are going to learn more about yourself and what you are capable of than you ever would have dreamed.

I'm sure you've heard that nursing school is hard. While I'm not going to disagree, I am going to challenge you to approach nursing school from a positive and hopeful mindset. Although nursing school will likely be one of the most challenging things that you have ever undertaken, you can sail through it with the right attitude and a good plan of action.

This book is designed to help you get organized, maximize your time, and follow a simple action plan for success. Every chapter is chocked full of easy-to-follow tips on everything from preparing for tests and clinicals to how to deal with instructor problems. I am going to provide you with an overview of what nursing school is like. I'll share the things I wish someone would have told me when I started school. Consider this book a roadmap for success and a guidebook on how to enjoy the journey.

Nursing students are busy people, so I did my best to get straight to the point in every chapter and give you the most important things that you need to know to not only survive but also thrive in your program. I concluded each chapter with a summary of the most important points and an action plan that you can follow to implement what you learned in the chapter.

Some of the chapters will be applicable to your journey right now such as, Chapter One, *Set Yourself Up to Succeed* (a chapter on how to get organized and prepared for the busy life of a nursing student) and Chapter Five, How to Maximize Your

Study Time and Ace Your Exams. Other chapters like Chapter Nine, *Everything You Need to Know About NCLEX* and Chapter Eleven, *Beyond Nursing School* will help you look forward to life after graduation and how to land your dream job. You'll want to refer to many of these chapters over and over again as you are working your way through school and beyond.

Here is a brief overview of what to expect in each chapter:

Chapter One — Set Yourself Up to Succeed starts off with seven tips to help you organize your life, your home, and your schedule to prepare to sail through nursing school. If you follow these seven simple tips, you will give yourself more productive time and less stress during the school year so that you can focus on being the best student you can be. Next, you will find the Essential Nursing Supplies Shopping List that you can use as a guide to what you really need to buy before you start school and what items are nice to have but not necessities.

Chapter Two — What to Expect in Nursing School: Five Things the Brochure Didn't Mention will give you insight into what nursing school is REALLY like (the good and the bad) and how to prepare yourself for the more challenging parts of school.

Chapter Three — A Day in the Life of a Successful Nursing Student and How to Structure Your Day begins with a look into what a successful nursing student's day is like from start to finish. Next, you will learn some tips on how to balance your busy life (family, relationships, work, etc.) with nursing school. Finally, I will give you a five-step plan to create your personal schedule that will set you up for a successful semester.

Chapter Four — How to Dominate Stress is a must-read chapter for any future nurse. Nursing is a high-pressure job. This chapter will teach you the fundamental concepts of stress and how to identify your stressors. Then you will learn how to dominate stress and test anxiety. Don't skip over this important chapter. Refer to it throughout the school year when you find yourself feeling stressed or on the verge of burn out.

Chapter Five — How to Maximize Your Study Time and Ace Your Exams is full of practical tips to help you study smarter, not just harder. You will learn the importance of short, focused study sessions and why they are more effective than long cramming sessions. You'll find sections here on notetaking, using practice questions, creating your own study guides, how to form a study group, and a lot more. I will even show you how to improve your memory and boost your brain function for maximum success.

Chapter Six — Simple Keys to Success is a short but important chapter that I wrote to share with you the things that I wished I would have known when I started school. I will cover things like the importance of self-care, how to set goals that motivate you, and why study groups are vital to your success.

Chapter Seven — Clinical Do's and Don'ts will give you straight to the point, practical tips on how to prepare for clinical work, what to do to make the most of this important time, and what not to do. Re-read these tips several times and commit them to memory so that you can be the Rockstar of your clinical group.

Chapter Eight — How to Stick it Out When Nursing School Gets Hard focuses on how to deal with instructor problems, bullies, and gender or racial discrimination. You'll learn how to deal with these difficult situations that are all too common in nursing school and the workplace.

Chapter Nine — Everything You Need to Know About NCLEX will show you how to register for your exam, how to prepare, and what to expect when you get to your testing center. You will learn my top nine tips to ace your NCLEX the first time.

Chapter Ten — Six Quick Tips to Enjoy Nursing School will show you how to make nursing school some of the best years of your life. Don't believe what you've heard; you can enjoy it! You'll read about things like why it's important to schedule fun into your schedule and how to celebrate the milestones on the way to getting your nursing degree.

Chapter Eleven — Beyond Nursing School will give you a peek into the life of a working nurse. You will learn about the different opportunities available to you as you graduate and how to land your dream job. This chapter will help you form an exciting vision for your future.

Resources for Your Journey is the final chapter, and here you will find the top books, podcasts, websites, blogs, social media pages, and YouTube video channels created for nursing students and working nurses. Utilize these helpful resources to learn more and stay motivated as you work to become the best nurse that you can be.

My hope is that this book will make your life as a nursing student easier and more enjoyable. It is meant to be used as a practical action guide to help you do your absolute best in your classes and clinicals. Follow through with your action steps, and you will have an advantage over the other students in your program.

If you have any questions or comments, I would love for you to email me at ContactUs@upgradeyourpath.com. If you found this book helpful, you can also leave a review on Amazon. Your review will help other nursing students find this book.
Let's get started on your nursing journey!

Chapter One
Set Yourself Up to Succeed

"As a nurse, we have the opportunity to heal the heart, mind, soul and body of our patients, their families and ourselves. They may forget your name, but they will never forget how you made them feel." Maya Angelou

Preparing for nursing school is a bit like preparing for a new baby. At the end of a pregnancy, women typically go through a nesting period when they prepare for a new pace of life. When you have a new baby, you have little time to clean your house, shop for groceries, or prepare meals, so women often spend the last month or so of their pregnancies stocking up on what they will need for those early months of adjustment. They will take care of any important matters that they might not have time to do after the baby comes.

If you want to sail through nursing school, you need to be prepared and organized. In this chapter, I will give you a lot of tips on how to get your life ready for this busy time so that you are not overwhelmed with trying to balance everything. These organizational tips will also help you build good habits that will serve you well during your nursing program and throughout your nursing career.

7 Tips to Prepare Your Life for Nursing School

The following tips will save you time and make your life easier when you get started on classes. Take some time in the weeks before nursing school starts to tackle these items. You'll be so grateful that you did.

There is a handy checklist at the end of the chapter that will help you get everything done.

Tip #1 Stock up on household essentials and buy in bulk. Over the next few months, you will have little time to make store runs if you run out of an important item. Make a list of the staple items that you will need over the next 2-3 months and stock up. Fill your cart with personal care items and pantry items that you know you will use. Bulk stores like Costco or Sam's Club are perfect for stocking up. Amazon or Walmart are other options. Take a look at your local flyers to find the best deals so that you can maximize your budget.

Here is a list of ideas to get you started.
- Personal Care Items:
- Deodorant
- Soap/bodywash
- Toothbrushes/Toothpaste
- Mouthwash
- Toilet paper
- Feminine care products
- Shampoo and conditioner
- Hair styling products
- Skincare products
- Makeup
- Razors/shaving cream
- Vitamins/supplements
- Pantry Items:

- Paper goods: Napkins and paper towels
- Household cleaners and laundry detergent
- Condiments: ketchup, mustard, mayonnaise, etc.
- Spices
- Coffee and Tea
- Easy to prepare foods like pasta, sauce, rice, beans, cereals, soups, etc.
- Pet food and pet supplies
- Bottled water
- Freezer Items:
- Fruits and vegetables
- Easy-to-prepare frozen meals

As you are choosing pantry items, try to stock up on a lot of healthy options. As a nurse, your body is your biggest commodity. Now is the time to build healthy habits of eating a lot of vegetables, fruits, organic grass-fed meats, and whole grains.

Save your list and reuse it every few months. Buying in bulk will save you a lot of time and money over the course of a school year.

Tip #2 Clean your house from top to bottom.
If you've ever tried to study in a messy room, you know how easy it can be to put off that 100 pages of reading that you don't feel like doing to fold the basket of laundry that's been sitting on your bed all week or clear the sink of dirty dishes from the night before.

Imagine coming home from your first day of nursing school to an immaculately clean home, sitting down to study at a neatly organized desk, and being able to focus on your reading without thinking about all of the things you need to get done around the house. That is our goal. And it's easier than you think.

Think of the week or two before nursing school as a time of spring cleaning. Go through your living space, room by room, and give it a thorough cleaning. Handle those tasks that you only do once and awhile like cleaning your fridge and vacuuming behind furniture. The cleaner you make it now, the easier it will be to maintain your home on a daily basis. (We'll talk about that more in tip #4.)

Tip #3 Declutter your home.
We all hold on to things that think we will use one day but never do. You will be amazed at how much neater your space will look if you take the time to clear out those items that you will realistically never use again.

As you are deep cleaning your home, divide the things that you don't use into three piles: things you can give away, things you can sell to help pay for nursing school supplies, or things you can throw away. If you have trouble deciding whether or not to keep something, ask yourself if you've used the item in the last six months. If the answer is no, let it go.

Utilize eBay or Craigslist to sell items that you don't use. This is a great way to pay for all of those expensive textbooks and supplies that we'll talk about later in the chapter. If you have a large number of items to sell and don't want to spend the time listing all of your items online, have a garage sale or split the profits with a friend or family member who enjoys listing items for sale online.

Tip #4 Create a simple 30-minute home upkeep routine.
Now that you have a clean and decluttered home, it's time to make a simple plan to keep it looking this way on a daily basis. You won't have time as a nursing student or a working nurse to spend hours cleaning your house. Now is the time to build good habits that will serve you for many years to come as you

are working 12-hour shifts and want to just kick back and relax on your days off.

You'll need to adjust the following home upkeep routine to your particular living situation. Depending on whether you live in a studio apartment by yourself, a four-bedroom house with your three kids to pick up after, or a cozy room in your parents' house, you may need anywhere from 10 minutes to 30 minutes per day to maintain your already clean living space.

The key to making this work is to do a little bit every day so that the housework doesn't pile up on you. This also won't work if you skipped over tip #3. If your house is full of clutter, you won't be able to keep your home clean using this simple routine.

Here are some items that you can get done in a 30-minute upkeep routine:

-       Make your bed as soon as you get out of it in the morning.
-       Throw a load of laundry in the washing machine in the morning and put it into the dryer when you get home.
-       Clear any dishes in your sink and wipe down the counters right after you eat your breakfast.
-       Choose one room in your house to vacuum or dust mop daily.
-       Also, vacuum dust from that same room after you clean the floor.
-       Make a habit of picking up two items in a room as you are getting ready to go to another room.
-       Give your bathtub and sink a quick wipe down every other morning after you shower.
-       After you brush your teeth, wipe down your mirror.

Depending on the size of your home or living space, cleaning for 15-30 minutes per day should be enough to maintain a decently clean home. You'll probably need to spend an extra hour or so per week to do larger tasks like mopping your kitchen floor or deep cleaning the tub.

Choose a time of day that works for you to fit this in or plan a couple of mini cleans during your daily routine. You can even listen to an audiobook or YouTube video to learn while you clean. (Check out the resources chapter to see what I recommend.) Figure out what routine works best for you and write it down to remind you until it becomes a part of your regular schedule.

Ask members of your household to help out with specific chores that are the most time-consuming. Let them know that you will especially need their help around the house while you are in school so that you have enough time to study. Keep chore charts in the house so that every member of the household remembers what they need to get done.

Tip #5 Fill your freezer with simple, healthy meals.
It is a wonderful feeling to come home to a home-cooked meal after a long day of classes, studying, and clinical hours. You can do this for yourself by filling your freezer with simple, healthy meals that you enjoy. When you get home, all you have to do is put your freezer meal in the oven and enjoy. If you are cooking for a family, this is an easy way to prepare good meals for your family with less stress.

The internet is full of easy freezer meal recipes. Choose a few that sound good to you and experiment until you find a rotation that you enjoy. Start filling your freezer with meals before school starts, and you can set yourself up nicely for your first month of school.

If you don't like to cook, find a friend or family member that does, and ask them to cook with you. Put on some music and make it a fun event. As you start school, this might be a fun activity to do with your study partners.

What Should You Cook?
Some stand-by freezer meal ideas are casseroles, chili, baked ziti, lasagna, stir-fry, stuffed peppers, stews, and soups. You can also freeze breakfast sandwiches and ready-to-go smoothie baggies for those mornings that you don't have time to cook a hot breakfast.

Here are a few tips to get you started:

Start simple
If you are new to making freezer meals, start small. Choose 2 or 3 meals to start with and simply cook a double batch. You don't need to spend hours in the kitchen your first time. If you get too ambitious the first time, you'll be less likely to make freezer meals again.

Make double dinners
If spending an afternoon cooking 2 or 3 meals is too much for you, you can simply plan to make a double batch of whatever you are making for dinner and freeze it. Do this just a few nights per week and you can fill your freezer with meals in no time.

Use gallon storage bags
Storing your freezer meals in gallon storage bags makes it easy to fill even a small freezer with several weeks of meals. If space isn't an issue, or you are feeding a large family, you can use foil baking pans or plastic storage bins made for freezing.

Label each container

Use permanent markers to label each meal with what it is and the date that you are freezing it. If you start to build up a large supply of freezer meals, do your best to consume the oldest meals first to avoid allowing good food to go to waste.

Avoid freezing recipes that include fried foods, mayo, yogurt, raw potatoes, or produce with a high-water content like cucumbers, lettuce, or melon.

Crockpot Cooking

An Instant Pot or crockpot can also be a lifesaver when you are trying to prepare meals as a busy student. Crockpots are wonderful because you can throw a bunch of healthy ingredients into the pot before you leave for school, turn it on low, and come home to a heavenly smell at the end of the day. Find a few simple recipes online, and experiment with the ones that sound the best to you.

Freezer Meal and Crockpot Recipe Websites:
AllRecipes.com
Delish.com
MyRecipes.com
SouthernLiving.com
TasteOfHome.com

A Quick Note About Your Diet

While we're on the topic of food, it's so important that you eat a healthy diet if you want to sail through nursing school. Make sure you eat balanced meals; a lot of nursing students make poor food choices and eat whatever they can grab to make more time to study. If you do this, you will find yourself gaining weight, having low energy, and experiencing skin issues such as acne.

During my associate degree program, I was eating in a horrible manner because all I wanted to do was study. I was focusing on this one semester — the very last semester — and I was stress-eating, and my skin took the beating. Learn from my mistakes, and fill your diet with a variety of vegetables, fruits, whole grains, lean meats, and fish. Drink lots of water to stay hydrated. You'll notice a difference in your energy and concentration in comparison to your friends who fill their diets with junk food and more coffee than water.

Tip #6 Automate your bills.
Take an hour or two now to put your finances on autopilot and save yourself a lot of time every month. This will also ensure that you never have to deal with trying to make an urgent payment because you forgot to pay a bill.

Most banks allow you to set up automatic payments from your checking account online. All you need is a copy of your current bills to enter the payment address, account number, and payment amount for each account. You can set up your bills to be paid based on when you are paid or when each bill is due. You can also set up automatic payments with each company individually, but this can be time-consuming.

It's also a good idea to have a portion of every paycheck automatically deposited into a savings account. Even if you only save $10 per paycheck, it's important to get into the habit of paying yourself something first. If you are in your 20s or 30s, don't wait to start saving. There are so many people in their 40s, 50s, and 60s who wish they'd started saving at your age. The compound interest can turn those small deposits into a nice little chunk of change over time.

Tip #7 Take care of anything you've been putting off or anything you can get done before school starts.
Sit down and make a list of anything that you've been putting off. Ask yourself what piece of unfinished business you can handle now so that it doesn't become an urgent distraction while you are focusing on school. Do you need to make an

important phone call? Is there some paperwork that you need to complete? Have you been putting off cleaning out your garage?

You can also look ahead in your schedule to see if there are any appointments that you might be able to get out of the way before school starts: an eye doctor appointment, dermatologist visit, vet appointment, car maintenance, your child's routine well-check, etc.

Now go through that list one by one and decide what you need to get done now and what can wait until the semester break. The simple act of writing things down and deciding when you will handle each item takes them out of your head so that you can focus on the tasks at hand.

Now that your life is organized, it's time to have fun shopping for school supplies.

Essential Nursing Supplies Shopping List
One of the most important things you need to do to prepare for nursing school is to purchase the right supplies. Your out-of-pocket expenses can add up quickly, so you need to know what is essential for you to have and what is nice to have but not an absolute necessity.
Before you go shopping, you need to take a good look at what your nursing program requires you to buy. Use this list as a guideline in conjunction with whatever your school requires of you.

Essential Shopping List

•   High-quality Stethoscope
One item you'll want to invest money in is a good stethoscope. You'll need to spend $75-$100 or more to get a good one but

remember that this will last you well into your nursing career. A quality stethoscope will also come with a strong warranty.

My favorite brand is Littman. This company offers a variety of high-quality stethoscopes at a lower cost than many other companies.

• Scrubs with Pockets (At least 2-3 sets)

Like most nursing students, you are probably excited to buy your first set of scrubs. Before you rush out to find your perfect set, you need to check with your nursing program to see if there are any criteria you need to meet.

Once you know what your school requires, be sure to bring your measurements with you to find the right fit. It's better to choose scrubs that are slightly big than too small. Scrubs can be unforgiving (especially white scrubs) if they are too tight.

Look for scrubs with pockets to carry around pens, guidebooks, notebooks, etc. Make sure to buy at least 2 or 3 sets so that you always have a backup if you get behind on your laundry. And it's always a good idea to keep a clean backup set with you during clinicals. Nursing can be a dirty job.

• Possible Must-Have Item: Lab Coat

Some programs will require you to wear a lab coat to clinicals. Check with your school to see if this is a requirement. If it is, be sure to put your name somewhere inside of your jacket to avoid getting it mixed up with another student's coat.

• The Right Underwear

If your school requires you to wear white scrubs, you will want to invest in several pairs of flesh- toned or white underwear. Ladies, it's a good idea to get seamless panties to avoid panty lines. You can also wear a white undershirt or camisole if you need extra coverage on top of your bra.

• Comfortable Nursing Shoes

Nursing students are on their feet a lot. You'll want to invest in the most comfortable and durable shoes that you can afford.

Again, check with your program on any requirements that you might need to meet. Whether you opt for nursing shoes or high-quality tennis shoes, be sure to choose a pair that is slip resistant to protect yourself from falls.

•   Compression Socks

Any working nurse will tell you that compression socks are a must. Don't wait until you start your career to invest in the health of your feet and legs. Compression socks help with blood circulation and prevent pain and fatigue from walking all day. You can also try compression sleeves if you prefer to wear regular socks.

•   Nursing Watch

Although some nurses will tell you that they don't use one (they use the wall clock), many programs will require you to buy a nursing watch and bring it to clinicals. This is an area where you can cut costs and buy an inexpensive analog watch with a second-hand value.

•   Clinical Bag

You'll want to have a dedicated bag for all of your clinical supplies so that you are never without the items that you need, and you don't waste time trying to track down what you need before class. You don't need to invest a lot of money on a bag. Choose something that fits all of your items in an organized way. It's a good idea to choose a water-resistant bag because you'll be putting your bag down on all kinds of questionable floors.

•   Lanyard or Badge Clip

Every nurse has a preference on whether to use a lanyard or a badge clip. Some nurses feel uncomfortable having a lanyard hanging around their neck that could potentially get caught on something or someone with all of the bending and reaching that nurses do. Others love it. Experiment with both and see what you like better.

Whether you go with a badge clip or lanyard, you'll want to invest in a good one that won't fall apart on you in the middle of a shift. I heard a story of one nurse whose cheap badge fell apart in the middle of the shift and the pieces hit the patient in her face. She was thankful that the pieces didn't harm her patient.

• Nursing Scissors

Nursing scissors are important for cutting tape, gauze, bandages, etc. This inexpensive purchase is a must-have for any nursing student.

• Possible Must-Have Item: Sphygmomanometer

Extra credit if you knew that a sphygmomanometer is another word for a blood pressure monitor. Just as important as a high-quality stethoscope is a good blood pressure monitor. You may not need to purchase this for your program, so if it's not on the required list, you can wait on this purchase and use the monitors that are provided for you.

• Clipboard

One staple that you'll want to have in your clinical bag is a clipboard to hold all of your papers and pens. You can purchase a nursing clipboard that has important information and charts printed on it which can be really helpful during clinicals and beyond. If you need to cut costs, a simple, sturdy wooden or plastic clipboard will work.

• Penlight

Penlights are essential for checking the pupils, mouth, or throat of your patients. It's also helpful for checking wounds in areas that are difficult to see. Because they are the size of a pen, they are convenient to carry around. This low-cost item is a must-have for your clinical bag.

• Pocket Notebooks

Purchase a few inexpensive pocket notebooks to keep with you during clinicals. These are handy to write down vital signs, important medical information, or care plan notes. Note: Never, ever write down patients' names or other identifying information for confidentiality reasons. You could get into serious trouble if you accidently leave your notebook somewhere.

• Pens

Get in the habit now of stocking up on clickable black pens. You will need them every day for the rest of your life as a nursing student and nurse. Although you may see all kinds of pen colors used by your fellow students, black is universally known as the right color to use on legal documents, so it's a safe bet.

• Sharpies

You will need sharpies for clinicals to write on medication stickers that go on IV bags and to mark dressing changes.

• Good Student Planner

A good student planner is essential to keeping track of all of the important dates, phone numbers, and information you'll need to remember during your program. You'll learn a lot more about planning systems later on in this book. Some students love having a physical planner to write things down, others will only use a digital planner. There is no right or wrong choice. Choose what works best for you.

• Highlighters

You will want to have a few highlighters on hand to mark any important information in your book while you are reading or in class. Mark anything that your teacher says will be on the test or anything that you need to study later.

Nice-to-Haves List

The following list of items are not necessary (unless your program requires them), but they can make your life a bit easier.

• Reliable Laptop or Tablet

A good laptop or tablet will make your life as a nursing student much easier, but if you are tight on money, a reliable desktop will do. Many students prefer taking notes in class on a laptop or tablet. It is also nice to have the ability to work on papers and presentations or access the internet while on campus or at your favorite coffee shop.

• Wheeled Backpack

While not a necessity, a wheeled backpack is an easy way to avoid back pain that can come from lugging around a backpack full of large textbooks everywhere. When you take good care of your body, you are protecting your future as a nurse.

• Nursing Starter Kit

You can purchase a "starter kit" that includes a lot of the equipment that you will use for examinations like a stethoscope, blood pressure monitor, nursing scissors, pen light, etc. These sets typically come in a nice bag that holds all of your supplies. If you opt to purchase a kit like this, be sure to research the quality of the equipment included in the bag. You don't want to waste your money on a cheap stethoscope or blood pressure monitor that you'll need to replace.

• Expensive Travel Mug

If you're going to take my advice and make your own coffee in the morning to bring with you, it's a good idea to purchase a large, high-quality travel mug that will keep your coffee hot. Cheap mugs often leave you with cold coffee by the time you get to your destination. A good mug will keep your coffee hot long enough for you to drink the whole thing.

Nursing School Preparation Checklist

Tip #1 — Stock up on household items and buy in bulk.

☐ Make a list of the essential items you'll need over the next 2-3 months.

☐ Look at local flyers to find the best deals and best places to shop for your items.

☐ Save your list for future bulk shopping trips every few months.

Tip #2 — Clean your house from top to bottom. Tackle tasks that you don't do on a regular basis.

Tip #3 — Declutter your home.

☐　　Go through each room in your home and place items into 3 piles: sell, giveaway, or throw away. Remember, if you haven't used it in the last six months, let it go.

☐　　List any items you want to sell on eBay or Craigslist. Plan a garage sale.

Tip #4 — Create a simple 30-minute home upkeep routine.

☐　　Make a list of items that you can get done in 15-30 minutes on a daily basis to keep your home clean. Put it on your schedule or post it on your fridge.

☐　　Schedule a longer 1-to-2-hour cleaning session once a week to handle bigger cleaning jobs like mopping the floor and scrubbing the bathtub.

☐　　Talk to family members or roommates about helping out while you are in school.

Tip #5 — Fill your freezer with simple, healthy meals.

☐　　Search the internet for freezer meals or crockpot recipes.

☐　　Buy your ingredients and galloon freezer bags or containers.

☐　　Experiment with new recipes until you find a rotation that you enjoy.

☐　　Plan a regular meal preparation day to stay organized or double batch your dinners a few nights per week.

Tip #6 — Automate your bills.

☐　　Gather all of your bills and set up automatic payments online through your bank or with each company individually.

☐　　Set up automatic deposits into your savings account. Even $10 savings from each paycheck is a good start.

Tip #7 — Take care of anything you have been putting off or anything you can get done before school starts.

☐　　Make a list of everything that you've been putting off and either do it now or schedule it.

☐   Look ahead at your upcoming semester and see if there is anything you can get done before school starts (car maintenance, medical appointments, vet care, etc.)

Essential Nursing Supplies Checklist

The following list is only a guideline. Remember to check with your program to see what you are required to buy and adjust this list as needed.
☐   High-quality Stethoscope
☐   Scrubs with pockets (At least 2-3 sets)
☐   Possible Must-Have Item: Lab Coat (check with your program)
☐   The Right Underwear (flesh-toned if you must wear white scrubs)
☐   Comfortable Nursing Shoes (nonslip)
☐   Compression Socks
☐   Nursing Watch
☐   Clinical Bag (Water resistant and large enough to fit all of your must-have items)
☐   Lanyard or Badge Clip
☐   Nursing Scissors
☐   Possible Must-Have Item: Sphygmomanometer (check with your program)
☐   Clipboard
☐   Pen Light
☐   Pocket Notebooks
☐   Pens (clickable, black)
☐   Sharpies
☐   Good Student Planner (physical or electronic)
☐   Highlighters

Nice-to-Haves:
☐   Reliable Laptop or Tablet
☐   Wheeled Backpack
☐   Nursing Starter Kit

☐   Expensive Travel Mug

Notes

Chapter Two

What to Expect in Nursing School: Five Things the Brochure Doesn't Mention

"When you're a nurse, you know that every day you will touch a life or a life will touch yours." Anonymous

Entering nursing school should be one of the most exciting times of your life. You are preparing to become skilled in a field that will allow you to make a big difference in the lives of thousands of people over your career. You will learn a lot about how to care for patients. You will also learn a lot about yourself and what you are made of. As any nurse will tell you, it is impossible to come out of school the same person you came in as.

This chapter will go over a few things that you might not expect about nursing school. I want to prepare you for these so that you are not caught off guard. I'll also give you some tips on how to deal with these unexpected, but common issues.

A. **Nursing school burnout is normal and preventable.**

With all of the demands put upon nursing students, it may not surprise you to hear that it is common to experience burnout at some point during your program. Out of all of the healthcare programs, nurses experience the highest rate of student burnout.

It is common for students to become overwhelmed with balancing their studies and clinical hours with other life commitments. The good news is, you can learn how to avoid burnout and what to do if you experience it. Self-care should be just as important to your daily schedule as attending classes and studying.

There are so many ways to deal with burnout and even avoid it all together. I cover all of these things in more detail throughout this book, but I'll list them quickly here:

How to Avoid Nursing School Burnout

1)   Take care of business. One 2010 study showed avoidance coping was the largest predictor of nursing school burnout (Chris Gibbons, Stress, Coping and Burn-out in Nursing Students, International Journal of Nursing Studies 2010). Avoidance coping is dealing with stress by putting off assignments or other important tasks in order to experience temporary relief of stress. The best way to avoid burnout is to be organized and disciplined. Putting off your assignments or study sessions until the last minute is a sure-fire way to be stressed.

2)   Take time to do something you love every day. Commit to finding one hour per day that is dedicated to something you

enjoy. Work on a hobby, read a novel, take an exercise class, work in your garden, go out with friends, watch a movie, or anything else that will allow you to forget about school and have fun. If you have a lot of other responsibilities on top of school and find it impossible to carve out one hour per day from your already busy schedule, try to give yourself at least one hour per week.

3)   Prioritize exercise to improve mental clarity, energy, and ability to deal with stress. One of the best ways that you can avoid stress and burnout is to make exercise part of your weekly routine. Healthy adults should get at least 150 minutes of cardio exercise (walking, jogging, playing basketball, swimming, cycling, dancing, etc.) every week. You should also include at least two sessions of resistance exercise like lifting weights or bodyweight exercises. Yoga or tai chi are also excellent exercises to keep your body and mind in shape.

4)   Find one or two friends in your nursing class to study with (and vent your frustrations to.) No one understands what you are experiencing as a nursing student quite like another nursing student. It is vital that you find one or two students in your program to whom you can vent your frustrations and receive encouragement on the hard days. Be careful to surround yourself with positive people and avoid spending a lot of time with negative people who complain all of the time. Spending your time with negative people will only add to your stress.

5)   Consider meditation. Taking even just 10 to 20 minutes to clear your mind of the day's worries and relax does wonders for your mental health. It's simple to learn, as it doesn't require any special equipment, and you can practice meditation anywhere. With regular practice, you'll walk through your day with a calmness and a greater ability to deal with stressors. If you have never tried meditation before, try taking a class or

download a guided meditation app (I personally like the Calm app).

If you are already experiencing burnout, there are many ways to deal with it:

1)   Talk to your instructor. Your instructors have been where you might be at any given moment, and they understand how demanding nursing school can be. Request a meeting with the instructor that you feel most comfortable expressing your feelings to and ask for advice on how to deal with what you are feeling.

2)   Keep a journal. Write down how you are feeling. Getting your feelings out of your head and putting them on paper can be therapeutic. You might even gain a better perspective on your situation by writing it all out.

3)   Vent to a fellow student. As I already mentioned above, you should seek out one or two friends in your program to study with and vent any frustrations to. If you're having a bad day, see if your friend will go for a walk with you or meet for coffee.

4)   Hit the gym or take a long walk. When you are feeling stressed or having a bad day, put on some inspiring music and get your body moving. Exercise releases proteins and hormones in your body that cause you to feel good and handle stress more effectively.

5)   Take a warm bath and read a good book or listen to music. Do something to relax, unwind, and forget about all of your obligations for an hour. After a good break, focus on a single important task that once it's completed will help you feel less overwhelmed.

6)   Listen to podcasts or read books that remind you of why you decided to become a nurse. I've included dozens of resources in the last chapter, including books, blogs, podcasts, and YouTube channels to keep you inspired to become the best nurse that you can be. Use these resources to help you stay motivated and encouraged throughout your nursing school journey.

Remember that you are not alone in your feelings. Just about every nursing student has experienced stress and burnout at some point during their program. You can handle this. Take it one day at a time, and don't give up.

B. **It will cost you more than you expect.**

Nursing school has more out-of-pocket expenses than most educational programs. As you already know, if you read Chapter 1, you'll need to invest in scrubs, comfortable shoes, clinical equipment, study tools, and lots of other items. And this doesn't even count tuition and textbooks. While I did my best to prepare you for what you'll need to buy, and what is nice to have, your program may require you to purchase other items that I didn't list in Chapter 1.

Here are some tips on how to save money for all of these extra expenses:

Find Lower Cost Textbooks
Textbooks can be a major expense for any student. Before you visit your campus bookstore, see if you can rent or buy your textbooks at a lower price online. Look at websites like Amazon and Student Rate Textbook. You can also call used bookstores in your area. If you know nurses who recently graduated nursing school, ask if they held on to their books and would be willing to sell them to you.

Create a Budget and Stick to It
If you don't have a personal budget, now is the time to create one. Set aside a certain percentage of your income for school expenses so that you don't have to struggle to scrape together funds for what you need.

Cook Meals at Home
Most students spend the majority of their income in coffee shops and fast food restaurants. You'd be amazed at how much money you can save every week by cooking the majority of your meals from home and investing in a nice coffee machine to bring your own coffee with you from home. Cooking from home also allows you to control the ingredients that you put in your food, so you can eat a healthier, more balanced diet.

C. **You will want to quit.**

No matter how prepared you are, or how positive your attitude is, there will probably come a time when you think about quitting. I don't want to be negative here, but I think that if you go into nursing school knowing that it is common to have these feelings, you will be better able to persevere through them and stick it out until graduation.
As I've already mentioned, nursing school requires a lot of study time and demanding clinical hours. You will be stretched farther than you have probably ever been stretched in your life. It is very common to doubt that you can meet all of the expectations that have been placed upon you.

When you do feel like quitting:
1)   Remember your ultimate goal. Sometimes it's easy to get so focused on the challenge of one class or one test that you lose sight of the big goal. Remind yourself that whatever you are working on right now is just a small part of getting to your big goal: to become an amazing nurse.

2)   Know that you are not alone. Take a moment to consider all of the nurses that have gone through nursing school and remember that you are just as capable of completing your program as they were.

3)   Talk to a mentor about what you are feeling. Ask to meet with a trusted instructor, tutor, or mentor. It's often helpful to get out of your own head and talk to someone else who understands how you feel and has successfully made it to where you want to be. A good mentor can help you gain a better perspective on your situation.

4)   Write down how you feel. If you don't want to talk with someone, it might help to write your feelings in a journal. Sometimes seeing your thoughts on paper helps you to see possible solutions you've never thought about before and gain a new perspective.

D. **Choose your friends wisely.**

One of the best things about nursing school is that you will develop a close group of friends that you will likely keep long after graduation. It is important to choose your friends wisely. Surround yourself with people who have good study habits and inspire you to be the best student you can be.

You've probably heard the saying that you are the sum total of your five closest friends. If you spend a lot of time with lazy, negative students, you will have a hard time making it through your program. There is nothing wrong with limiting the time you spend with people who drag you down. Remember your priorities and set yourself up for success by spending time with people who push you to do your best every day. Be the friend that you want to be by encouraging your friends and they will likely return the favor.

E. **You will need to get used to foul smells…quickly.**

Some nursing students are surprised with how difficult it is to get accustomed to dealing with the foul smells that they are exposed to on a daily basis in clinicals. Vomit, infections, urine, feces, and c-diff. are all common occurrences on a nursing shift, so you'll need to learn how to handle these odors without offending your patients.

Here are a few quick tips to learn how to deal with foul smells:
1.   Prepare yourself for potential smells by reading the patient's chart before you walk into the room. If you know ahead of time that the patient has a potentially smelly infection, it'll be easier to deal with.
2.   Place a bit of lavender essential oil on your wrist and use it to combat any smells when you need it.
3.   Wear mint-flavored chap stick or chew mint-flavored gum to help counterattack smells.
4.   Focus on empathizing with your patient. Place yourself in your patient's shoes. He or she is likely embarrassed and doesn't want to be in that room any more than you do. Do everything you can to make them feel comfortable.

Chapter Summary and Putting it into Action

Summary
Five Things that the Nursing School Brochure Doesn't Tell You
1)   Nursing school burnout is normal and preventable. Self-care should be just as important to your daily schedule as attending classes and studying.
2)   It will cost you more than you expect. Nursing school has more out-of-pocket expenses than most educational programs. Use the tips in this chapter to save money.
3)   You will want to quit. When you feel like quitting, talk to a mentor, write down your feelings, and remember your ultimate goal.

4) Choose your friends wisely. If you spend a lot of time with lazy, negative students, you will have a hard time making it through your program. Spend time with positive, hardworking students who encourage you to be at your best.

5) You will need to get used to foul smells quickly. Many nursing students are surprised at the amount of foul smells that they need to get used to on a daily basis.

Put it into Action
Tips to Avoid Nursing School Burnout:
- Take care of business: Procrastinating on assignments and studying is the fastest way to get burned out. Don't put off studying until the last minute.
- Do something you love every day: Try to carve out an hour every day to do something that you enjoy.
- Exercise regularly: Regular cardiovascular exercise and resistance training helps you deal with stress. Strive for 150 minutes of cardio and 2 days of resistance training every week.
- Find one or two friends to study with and vent your frustrations to when needed: It's important to surround yourself with positive people and to be positive yourself. Occasional venting is healthy.
- Consider meditation: Just 10 to 20 minutes of daily meditation can help you deal with stress easier and be a more peaceful person. Try guided meditation apps like Calm.

Tips to Deal with Burnout: If you are dealing with burnout, here are a few ways to deal with it.
- Talk to your instructor about how you are feeling.
- Write down your thoughts in a journal to gain a better perspective.
- Vent to a fellow student.
- Take a long walk or hit the gym.
- Take a warm bath and read a good book or listen to music.

-       Listen to a nursing podcast or book (not a textbook) that reminds you of why you decided to become a nurse. See the resources section in the back of this book for ideas.

Tips to Save Money on Nursing School Costs:
-       Find lower cost textbooks online or call used bookstores. Rent books online or from your learning center.
-       Budget for school supplies each semester. Put a little away from each paycheck to make it easier.
-       Cook meals at home. Bring coffee from home in the morning.

Tips to Deal with Foul Smells:
-       Read your patient's chart before you enter the room to prepare yourself for any potential foul smells.
-       Put lavender essential oil on your wrist to help you deal with any smells throughout the day.
-       Wear mint-scented chap stick or chew mint-flavored gum.
-       Empathize with your patient. Remember they are probably embarrassed.

Notes

Chapter Three

A Day in the Life of a Successful Nursing Student and How to Structure Your Day

"To do what nobody else will do, a way that nobody else can do, in spite of all we go through; that is to be a nurse." ~ Rawsi Williams

My goal is to give you an inside look into what it is like to be a nursing student so that you know what to expect and how to plan for success. In this chapter, you'll learn what a day in the life of a nursing student is like. I'll give you some helpful tips on how to balance your school and study schedule with the rest of your life. Finally, you will learn how to structure your day for success in school and life.

A Day in the Life of a Successful Nursing Student

6:00am Time to wake up.
Drink 16 ounces of water first thing in the morning to rehydrate. I'll also eat a banana or protein bar before getting ready to workout.

6:15 am Throw on some workout clothes and take a relaxing walk to start the day with a burst of energy. Getting a workout done in the morning ensures that it gets done.

7:00am After stretching and spending a few minutes meditating, it's time to shower, change, and finish getting ready for the day.

Pack Lunch and School Bag and Make Coffee to Go: Pack a good lunch with plenty of healthy snacks to avoid wasting money on fast food. Fill a large travel mug with coffee to save money and time going to the coffee shop.

Review today's schedule and pack a school bag with everything I need for the day. Time to get to class.

8:30am Class time or clinical hours depending on the day of the week.

11:30am On class days, I take a lunch break outside with friends. Lunch break is much shorter on clinical days and times will vary.

12:30pm Prepare for the next class.

1:00pm Next lecture or more clinical hours after a short break.

3:00 pm Take a short snack break before meeting a study group at the library. We are preparing for a big exam at the end of the week.

5:00 pm Go home and put one of my homemade freezer meals into the oven. Enjoy a relaxing dinner.

5:45 pm Take an hour to do something I enjoy doing.

6:45 pm Study a few more hours using the Pomodoro technique (25 minutes of focused study and 5-minute breaks in between).

9:45 pm Call my best friend to make plans to meet for dinner after my exam on Friday.

10:00 pm Get ready for bed and enjoy a full 8 hours of sleep.

While this is a fictitious account of a nursing student's day, I included this schedule to show you that it is possible to create a balanced day around a busy class, clinical, and study schedule. Of course, your schedule will look different depending on your commitments. Your clinical schedule may also vary from week to week, so it's important to stay flexible.

If you have a spouse and children, or a part-time job, you will need to schedule studying around everything else you have going on. Don't worry, I will help you create a foundational routine that covers all of your priorities and allows for the flexibility of a nursing student's hectic schedule.

How to Balance Nursing School with Life

"Don't confuse having a career with having a life." — Hillary Clinton

Balancing nursing school and the rest of your life requires preparation and intention. You need to make time for classes, studying, projects, and clinical hours, as well as family, friends, exercise, hobbies, and self-care. Achieving this balance while you are in school will make it much easier to maintain a strong work-life balance when you are a busy working nurse.

Here are a few tips to help you find the right balance for you.

Create Your Quiet Space

One of the things that helped me make it so far through school is creating a space for myself. You can set a place in your home that you know is your quiet area where you won't be disturbed, and your family knows when you're in that area that you are doing your homework and not to be bothered. Not only will this help you to focus on your schoolwork, but it will help you to put away your schoolwork when you need to spend time with your loved ones or enjoy your life outside of school. Although it might feel like nursing school is taking over your life at times, you don't have to let it. Making time and space for both school and relationships will help you avoid burnout and enjoy your time in school much more.

Humorous story: when I was in the associate degree nursing program, I had two little boys that were 11 months apart, so that was a lot of work in itself, and most times, they didn't understand their mummy is doing her homework. But I would hide in the closet in my bedroom hoping they don't come over and find me. Then one day, one of my sons found me, and he said, "Why are you in here?" I told him I was wondering the same thing. "Why are you in here, too?" I replied. It was a funny moment. I was determined to study. Always have your own space!

Remember You Are Doing It for Them
On the topic of children, if you are a parent like me, your children might have a difficult time adjusting to spending less time with you. Help your child cope by creating a special routine that you do together on a regular basis to remind them that they are your priority: read a book every night together before bed, walk together after dinner, cook breakfast together on Saturday mornings, have a family game night on Friday nights, etc. Ask your child what he or she would like to do with you, then put it on your calendar so that you follow through.

There will be days that it will be difficult to be away from your children. Remind yourself that you are sacrificing now to create a better life for them. School will not last forever, and you will soon get to celebrate all of your hard work with your children. Best of all, your example of sacrifice and hard work will make a lasting impression on your children that will help them to become successful at reaching whatever goal they set out to achieve.

Plan to Make Time for Relationships
"Failure of your company is not failure in life. Failure in your relationship is." — Ev Williams
Make time for your family and other important relationships by including this in your schedule. Even if you can only spare 20 minutes after you return from school, it will be time well spent. Prioritizing time with loved ones makes it easier for them to understand the goals that you are working on and why you

are so busy. If you're married or have children, it's important that you make it clear that although you may need to spend less time with them, you are working so hard to provide a better life for all of you. Spend time with your family no matter how huge the pressure is.

Make Your Own Schedule for Success in Four Easy Steps

Step #1 — Start with your priorities in mind.
As I have already touched upon, it's important to keep a balanced schedule to avoid overwhelm, stress, and burnout. Your schedule should include your classes and time for studying, as well as time for exercise, time with family, and fun events. Although you will need to make some temporary sacrifices while you are in school, proper planning should allow you to still live a well-balanced life.

Before you start making your schedule, write down your priorities. What are the most important things that you need to focus on in your life on a weekly basis? Obviously, nursing school will be near the top of your list for the next few months. Other priorities might be a spouse, children, health, a job, your spiritual life, a hobby, etc. Write your priorities down and refer to this list as you create your master schedule in Step 3.

Step #2 — Choose your method of schedule keeping.
Before we begin making your master schedule, you need to choose where you will keep your schedule. This can be a student planner, a binder, a smartphone, a computer software, or a large whiteboard in your home. The best answer is the method that you know you will use. If you know that you won't carry around a paper planner, but you always have your phone with you, a Google calendar on your smartphone might work best. If you love writing things down, a physical planner is probably your best bet. If you like being able to see your schedule written out on a wall calendar or whiteboard in your

home, you should do that, and consider taking a picture of your schedule to carry around in your phone so that you can access your schedule on the go.

I personally like to print out my schedule and to-do lists so that I can cross things off as I get them done. This helps me stay organized and not forget important tasks. If you are not sure what works best for you, start with what you think will work best and experiment until you find the right fit.

Step #3 — Build your master schedule.
Once you've made a list of your priorities and chosen a schedule-keeping method, it's time to create a master schedule. A master schedule is a basic outline of what your typical week will look like with all of your priorities attended to. You can use this schedule as the foundation of each week's schedule and adjust it to fit what you have going on in a particular week.

To make your master schedule, go day by day through a typical week, and write down everything you need to do from the time you wake up in the morning until bedtime (like the example at the start of this chapter). Be sure to fill in all of your classes, time to study, study groups, family time, work schedule, meals, household chores, exercise, and any other obligations you have. Refer to your priorities list and make sure that you are making time for the things that are most important in your life.

Step #4 — Plan to plan.
Extremely productive people make weekly planning time a priority. Choose a day and time out of the week, like Sunday afternoons at 3pm, and make this your weekly planning session. Take out your syllabi, work schedule, and any other calendars you have, and look at what you have coming up for that week. Create your schedule using your master schedule as the foundation. If you have a big test coming up, you may need to postpone going out with your friends this week to get some

extra studying in. If you have an important family event coming up on a night when you would usually study for 3 hours, see where you can find an additional 3 hours in your schedule on another day so that you can attend the event.

Taking just 15-20 minutes to look at your upcoming week and make any needed adjustments to your schedule will help you keep a balanced schedule based on your priorities and help you to stay on top of upcoming tasks and events.

How to Find Time to Study When You're a Parent
What do you do when you've plugged in all of your responsibilities into your master schedule and there's not enough hours in the day to study? I understand how hard it is to balance nursing school and being a wife and mother. Here are some tips to help you find extra time to study.

Wake Up Early or Stay Up Late
One of easiest (and hardest if you're a night owl) ways to add on one or two more hours to your day is to wake up before your children. It might be difficult to begin waking up early if you are used to waking up with your children, but your body will typically adjust after consistently waking up at the same time every day for a few weeks. The key is to make sure that you go to sleep early enough to get at least 7-8 hours of sleep so that you are well-rested.

If waking up one or two hours before your children sound like an impossible idea, you might want to schedule your study sessions for after your children go to sleep. If you choose to go this route, make sure that this is a time of day when you actually have the energy and ability to concentrate on your studies. If you are exhausted by the end of the night, you may want to consider simply reviewing your notes for a few minutes each night, going to sleep early, and waking up for early morning study sessions.

Tap into Your Support System
If you have small children who need a lot of your time, talk to your spouse, another family member, or a close friend and ask for help. Even just one evening a week of help can make a difference in your study schedule.

Paying for a few hours of childcare on a weekly basis or only on the weeks when you might need some extra study time is also an option if your budget allows. I've also heard of student-moms who share the cost of a babysitter during their weekly group study sessions.

Encourage Your Kids to Study with You
For very small children, create a special "study bag" just for them with toys and books that they only get to play with while you are studying. Fill the bag with things like small books, blocks, coloring books and crayons, art paper, buttons, string, stickers, and anything else that might interest him or her. Periodically switch out the items to keep it interesting.

For school-age children, you can make this their study time and encourage them to focus on a hobby or new interest like studying space exploration or making friendship bracelets. Not only will this give you extra focused time to study, but it will help your kids see that studying is a discipline that requires regular, focused time.

Utilize Small Windows of Time
We all have small windows of 15-30 minutes throughout our day that can be better utilized. Carry your study notes or flashcards with you to fit in some extra study time while you are waiting for your kids at sports practice, sitting under the dryer at the hair salon, taking public transportation, waiting in

the carpool line, or standing in line at the grocery store. All of these small windows of time can add up by the end of a day.

Chapter Summary and Putting it into Action

Summary
With some careful planning, you can create a master schedule that will help you cover all of your priorities. Successful students make time for sleep, exercise, self-care, and relationships. Being a good student does not mean that you can't live a balanced life.

How to Balance Nursing School with Life
☐   Create a quiet space to study. Not only will this help you to focus on your schoolwork, but it will also help you to put away your schoolwork when you need to spend time with your loved ones or enjoy your life outside of school.
☐   Remember that you are sacrificing time with your family to make a better life for them.
☐   Plan time for relationships. Even if you can only spare 20 minutes after you return from school, it will be time well spent. Prioritizing time with loved ones makes it easier for them to understand the goals that you are working on and why you are so busy.

Putting it into Action
Make Your Own Schedule for Success in Five Easy Steps
Step #1 — Start with your priorities in mind.
Before you start making your schedule, write down your priorities. What are the most important things that you need to focus on in your life on a weekly basis?

Step #2 — Choose your method of schedule keeping.

Choose where you will keep your schedule. This can be a student planner, a binder, a smartphone, a computer software, or a large whiteboard in your home. The best answer is the method that you know you will use.

Step #3 — Build your master schedule.
Write down everything you need to do from the time you wake up in the morning until bedtime. Be sure to fill in all of your classes, time to study, any study groups, family time, work schedule, meals, household chores, exercise, and any other obligations you have. Refer to your priorities list and make sure that you are making time for the things that are most important in your life.

Step #4 — Plan to plan.
Choose a day and time out of the week and make this your weekly planning session. Take out your syllabi, work schedules, and any other calendars you have, and look at what you have coming up for that week. Create your schedule using your master schedule as the foundation.

How to Find Time to Study When You're a Parent
Parents of small children might need to get creative to find enough time to study.
•   Wake up early to study, or study after the kids are in bed.
•   Tap into your support system. Ask family members and friends to help out so that you can study.
•   Encourage your kids to study with you. Create a "study bag" for small children toys and books that they only play with while you are studying. School-age children can use this time to focus on learning about something new or working on a hobby.
•   Utilize small windows of time. Carry your study notes or flashcards with you to fit in some extra study time while you

are waiting for your kids at sports practice, taking public transportation, or waiting in the carpool l

Notes

Chapter Four

How to Dominate Stress and Anxiety

"Nurse, just another word to describe a person strong enough to tolerate everything and soft enough to understand everyone."
Anonymous

"Everyone else gets to go out, go to the bars, go on dates, workout, go to the lake, but I am just sitting here trying to pass nursing school," says a worn-out student from clinical. It may seem like you are under constant stress as a nursing student while everyone else is enjoying life. Stress can cause you to forget the big picture of what you are working so hard to achieve. I succeeded in learning how to dominate stress, and you can too.

It is common to experience stress; we are all wired to handle the stress of our daily lives, but no one told us to settle for it. So, it's not the stress that negatively affects us; it's our response to it. STRESS is frequently described as being overpowered or suppressed; however, stress is our body's natural response to dealing with a perceived danger.

In the proper context, stress can be helpful. Some pressure can be valuable now and again in nursing school. It can deliver a lift that gives the push needed to pass tests or meet assignment due dates. When not dealt with properly, stress can cause both physical and mental problems and paralyze us rather than propel us forward.

Then we have STRESSORS, and I call them "the Marauders," they slink in like a thief in the night to cause stress. I'll share with you my experience with stress and anxiety and how I overcame them. Hopefully this will help you to spot the stressors in your life and learn how to deal with stress so that it is helpful and not harmful.

Stress Throws You Off Your Game
I had so many things going on in my life during nursing school, that I was overwhelmed and stressed out. I can recall a time while I was in my vocational nursing program when I got furious after someone shared bad news with me right before the start of a test. I became so confused that I forgot everything that I studied, and I failed the test.

I had prepared really hard for this test and was sure that I was going to pass it before I heard this awful news. I knew the material, but my mind wasn't clear, and I had no time to calm down or go out and meditate before the test began. I wasn't able to deal with the stressor (this bad news) before going into my test. Here's why you need to focus on stressors; they literally invade your mind and throw you off your game.

"To be a champion, you have to learn to handle stress and pressure. But if you've prepared mentally and physically, you don't have to worry." These are Harvey Mackay's words, but many would say, "easier said than done," right? No! It's our choice! We were made to handle stress properly.

The What, How, and Why of Stress?
In *The Art of War*, Sun Tzu wrote, "If you know the enemy and know yourself, you need not to fear the result of a hundred battles..." You might say, "What has The Art of War got to do with stress?" Well, if you don't see stress as a threat, you may succumb to it, and I'm sure you're growing tired of how it can mess up your day. Before we get into how to manage stress and stressors, we'll look at three questions: WHAT does stress do to me? HOW do I end up stressed? And WHY?

WHAT does it do? It does damage to your body and messes with your mind.
Stress can cause physical effects like fatigue, illness, stomach upset, sleep issues, pain in the chest, muscle pain, etc. Mood effects are common such as, frustration, restiveness, diminished motivation, overwhelming feelings, worries, etc. And behavioral effects like stress eating, social abstinence, outrages, and drug abuse, etc. are often the result of unchecked stress. The list of the negative effects of stress go on and on.

HOW do you end up in such a situation? Here's where we need to focus on stressors.
Just know that anything that puts excessive demands on you can cause stress. Anything from trying to balance a busy schedule of clinicals and lectures along with a growing family, financial worries, health problems, broken relationships, and worries about the future can all become stressors. It is important to realize what your stressors are so that you can better deal with them. Sometimes we get so used to being chronically stressed that we don't even take a minute to realize what the root cause is. When you are feeling stressed, ask yourself how you got to this point.

WHY? Not all stress originates from things that transpire in our lives.

A lot of our stress is self-initiated. When we allow ourselves to focus too long on problems instead of solutions or make an issue bigger than it has to be, we cause our own stress. At times we can even create problems that are not even there. When we worry about the "what ifs," instead of focusing on the truth of the matter, we can create unnecessary stress.

There is good news: humans have the gift of controlling their thoughts; oh yes, you can. So, let's go on to discuss how to deal with these interlopers!

Dominating Stress

Someone once said, "Adopting the right attitude can convert a negative stress into a positive one." There will always be dark days, but everyone has the potential to train their mind to better handle stress. After some time and practice, you can dominate stress and use it to your advantage.

When you have stress at school, or you are letting your instructors and classmates upset you, or you're stressing about your grades, it can alter your mood. Before I knew how to identify my stressors and deal with stress, I would often take it out on my family who had absolutely nothing to do with it. I call it "Kicking-the-Dog" syndrome. When you can't kick the individual or the situation that you are annoyed with, you proceed to kick another person who can't defend themselves.

This can happen in marriages. One person is dealing with a lot of stress in school or work and takes it out on their spouse without truly understanding what they are doing. Because the stressed-out spouse doesn't understand stressors or how to properly deal with their stress, their partner assumes that their spouse hates them for no reason. As you can imagine, this will lead to constant arguing and can easily end in separation, if not dealt with properly.

I know that may seem like an extreme example, but it is all too common with nursing students considering all of the demands on our lives. This doesn't have to be your story. I am going to share several tools that you can use to keep stress from destroying your life.

Try Meditation: One thing I did that helped a lot during nursing school was to step away for at least 10 minutes and clear my mind or meditate. I use this app called "Calm" which has any type of meditation you can think of for any scenario. I like using guided meditations because it can be difficult in the heat of a stressful situation to calm down on your own. Many studies show that regular meditation can improve your body's natural ability to deal with stress and improve your overall mood even when you are not meditating.

Write Down Your Stressors: It is imperative that you understand your stressors in order to handle stress properly. One approach is to write down all of the potential stressors that could be at the root of your stress: an upcoming exam, clinicals, your boyfriend, debt, worries about not finding a job after graduation, etc.

Once you write this down, you'll probably notice that your stressors are more about how you are dealing with any problems you might be facing than the actual problem. When you identify the stressors, you can start looking for productive solutions like meditating or exercising to release stress, creating a plan to deal with a difficult problem, or talking to a close friend to get a better perspective, etc.

Be Positive: Positive people are often better at handling stress because they know that things will eventually work for the best. Regardless of your current mindset, you can practice being a more positive person until it eventually becomes a part of your default thinking.

One way to rehearse a positive outlook is to read daily affirmations out loud to yourself. Tell yourself things like, "today is going to be a great day," or "I am highly intelligent, and I will ace all of my exams," or "I was created to be an excellent nurse, so I can handle any challenge that I encounter in clinicals."

Another easy way to become a more positive person is to surround yourself with other positive people. Limit your time with people who complain a lot and seem to drain your energy after spending time with them.

Seek Help: Try not to feel like you need to make sense of your stress by yourself. Look for help and backing from family and companions, regardless of whether you feel the need for somebody to hear you out or not. Talking with someone can take your mind off the stress and ease tension. Getting someone else's perspective on your situation might even help you see that you are blowing your current situation out of proportion.

Take Control: Having a stressful shift? Just relax and breathe. Stress can be activated by an issue that may superficially appear to be difficult to settle. Figuring out how to discover answers for your problems will enable you to feel more in charge. After you take a minute to relax and breathe, you'll be in a better place to come up with solutions. Remember that our brains are designed to find with solutions to problems. If you get really stuck, ask for advice from a trusted mentor or friend.

Study to Build Confidence: You might be surprised to know that nursing school tests are just like any other academic test. The only reason we feel like it's rocket science and get stressed out over them is that we are not prepared. It took some time before I realized this myself. A nursing student once told me, "Finals week is literally every week in nursing school. We

haven't gone a week without a major test this entire semester."
Although she was right, it's important to remember that these
tests are designed to prepare us for the important work of
caring for people and saving lives. Nursing programs have
been around for centuries, and hundreds of thousands of
people have passed. You can too!

Visualize: Visualization is a valuable stress management
method. World-class athletes use visualization to prepare for
big games by visualizing themselves performing at a high level.
You can use it to decrease test pressure or become a better
student by envisioning yourself accomplishing your objectives
with great success.

Take a couple of minutes every day and picture what you
would like to occur, whether it's acing a test, performing a
perfect procedure, being a better dad, or simply being a more
positive person.

Beat Test Anxiety
Most nursing students, regardless of how much they prepare,
experience some form of test anxiety. While a touch of pressure
can motivate you to study harder, for certain students, test
anxiety can be crippling to the point that it severely alters a
student's academic career. Rest assured that test anxiety is very
common among nursing students, and you can overcome it
with some very simple tools.

We have already covered some of these tools in this section:
• Meditate on a daily basis
• Talk with a friend or fellow student about your worries
• Keep a journal
• Join a study group

Visualization is a powerful way to overcome test anxiety. The
week before your test, spend 5-10 minutes imagining yourself

calmly acing your test. See yourself sitting in your classroom feeling extremely prepared and knowing the answer to every question. If you have never tried visualization before, this might sound strange, but it works. Give it a try.

Study early. You can also combat test anxiety by starting to study for an exam as early as possible. Take a look at your syllabus at the beginning of the semester and plan to start studying for each exam as early as possible. Avoid cramming for exams at the last minute, this will only increase your anxiety.

Use practice tests. Another way to overcome test anxiety is to take practice tests. If you are part of a study group, put together practice exams for one another and take the exams as part of your study time. Simulating exams like this is a smart way to overcome anxiety because you can put yourself under pressure that is similar to what you experience on exam day. I will go into this technique in much more detail in Chapter Five.

Use relaxation techniques. Try relaxation techniques during the exam like taking deep breaths and relaxing your muscles. Take a break to walk around and get a drink of water. You can also try putting a little lavender essential oil on your wrist to help you stay calm.

Rest and eat well before your exams. Get a full 7-8 hours of sleep the night before your test, and eat a good, healthy breakfast. Studies show that sleep deprivation and poor eating habits inhibit our ability to handle stress and recall information, so staying up all night to study before a test is one of the worst things that you can do.

If none of these techniques work for you, get help from your instructors or your learning center. Anxiety is a very common problem, and you should never feel too embarrassed to ask for help. Unfortunately, many students suffer in silence because they think that asking for help is weak. On the contrary, asking for help can be one of the strongest things you do.

Chapter Summary and Putting it Into Action

Summary
What, How, and Why of Stress

What: Stress is our body's natural response to a perceived danger. When left unchecked, it can cause physical problems like fatigue, illness, chest pain, and muscle pain. Stress can also impact your concentration, motivation, and ability to recall information.

How: Stress can be caused by extreme demands that are placed on our lives such as: balancing school with other large obligations, financial issues, broken relationships, health issues, and worries about the future. It is important to recognize your stressors so that you can come up with solutions to combat them.

Why: A lot of our stress is self-initiated. When we allow ourselves to focus too long on problems instead of solutions or make an issue bigger than it has to be, we cause our own stress.

Put What You Learned into Action

Dominate Stress
There always will be dark days, but everyone has the potential to train their mind to better handle stress and use it to their advantage.

Try Meditation: Studies show that regular meditation can improve your body's natural ability to deal with stress and improve your overall mood even when you are not meditating.

Write Down Your Stressors: Write down all of the potential stressors that could be at the root of your stress. You'll probably notice that your stressors are more about how you are dealing with any problems you might be facing than the actual problem.

Be Positive: Read daily affirmations out loud to yourself. Tell yourself things like, "today is going to be a great day," or "I am highly intelligent, and I will ace all of my exams."

Seek Help: Look for help and support from family and companions, regardless of whether you feel the need for somebody to hear you out or not. Talking with someone can take your mind off the stress and ease tension.

Take Control: After you take a minute to relax and breathe, you'll be in a better place to come up with solutions. Remember that our brains are designed to come up with solutions to problems.

Study to Build Confidence: Stress in school is often caused by being unprepared and cramming for exams. Avoid stress by staying on top of your assignments and maintaining a regular study schedule.

Beat Test Anxiety
- Meditate on a daily basis
- Talk with a friend or fellow student about your worries
- Keep a journal
- Join a study group
- Visualize yourself calmly acing your exams
- Start studying early for your exams so that you are well prepared
- Don't cram for tests, it will cause more anxiety
- Use practice tests to simulate the pressure you will feel during an exam

• Use relaxation techniques like deep breathing, relaxing your muscles, or taking a break to clear your mind
• Try putting a little lavender essential oil on your wrist to stay calm
• Get a full 7-8 hours of sleep and eat a good breakfast before your test
If none of these techniques work for you, get help from your instructors or your learning center.

Notes

Chapter Five

How to Maximize Your Study Time and Ace Your Exams

"America's nurses are the beating heart of our medical system."
President Barack Obama

There are entire books written on various study methods alone. I've included a list of a few good ones in the resources chapter at the back of the book. This chapter is meant to provide you with some solid tools to help you maximize the time you spend studying and recall more information on your exams. You will also learn different methods of notetaking, how to avoid distractions while studying, and when to seek tutor assistance. At the end of the chapter, you'll learn why it's important to discipline your mind and how to improve your memory and recall.

Pomodoro Technique
The Pomodoro Technique is a simple, yet powerful way to maximize your study time, stay focused, and make studying more enjoyable. Entrepreneur Francesco Cirillo invented this technique in the late 1980s as a university student. He named

the technique after a tomato-shaped timer (*pomodoro* is Italian for tomato) that he used to track 25-minute study intervals.

Cirillo wrote a book called The Pomodoro Technique, but you don't have to read the book in order to understand and use the concept.

1) Break down one larger task into smaller tasks that you can get done in short, 25-minute intervals.

For example, you can break 100 pages of reading down into 4 sessions of 25 pages each.

2) Set your timer for 25 minutes and focus your complete attention on one task until the timer goes off. You can use an old-fashioned timer, your watch, or your phone.

3) Take a 5-minute break from your task. This is a good time to get up from your study space and walk around. Maybe do a few jumping jacks or pushups to get your blood circulating. Don't check your phone unless you're disciplined enough to put it away at the conclusion of your 5-minute break.

4) Start your timer again for another 25 minutes and get started on your next pomodoro. Again, give your full attention to one task for the entire 25 minutes.

5) Take a 15-to 30-minute break after every 3 or 4 pomodoros. This is a good time to check your phone, take a short walk, get some fresh air, or do something else that refreshes you.

The key to making this work is that you devote 100% of your attention to your task for the full 25-minute sprint. If you are interrupted, that does not count as a full pomodoro. You need to restart it. Turn off your TV and music, put your phone in another room, and focus your complete attention on the task at hand until that timer goes off.

If someone interrupts you during one of your 25-minute sessions, politely let them know that you are studying and agree on a better time to talk. Nobody will respect your time if you don't, so it's important to let those in your life know that you take your study time seriously.

This technique is powerful because it allows you to operate from a place of rest. By taking a 5-minute break every 25 minutes to get refreshed, you are giving yourself the best opportunity to approach each pomodoro with more motivation, focus, and creativity.

Millions of people use this technique to be more effective in their studies and work day. Try it yourself and you will see why it is so popular. There are a ton of phone apps you can experiment with like Focus Keeper and Flora that include a timer and a to-do list for you to keep track of your pomodoros. You can also try desktop software like Tomighty that allows you to customize your work and break periods.

Notetaking Methods and Tips
In order to sail through nursing school, you need a method for taking notes that works for you. Messy, unorganized notes will make it close to impossible for you to study from. Developing strong notetaking and organizational skills as a student will serve you well as a working nurse, so do yourself a favor and master this skill now.

I am going to present three different methods for you to choose from. Consider what will work best for you or try each one and see what you like best. The best method is the one that is easiest for you to implement in class and study from.

Take Notes on Lecture Slides
Many instructors will provide links to the slides that they will use during their lecture. You can print the slides and take notes

right on the page. This makes it easy for you to review what you will be covering and follow along in class. Mark anything that your instructor tells you will be on the exam and any information that he or she seems to emphasize in the lecture. You can even use a highlighter to mark important slides.

Purchase a sturdy binder, dividers, and a three-hole punch so that you can organize your notes by class, in the order that you created them.

Use Technology

A lot of students prefer to use a laptop or tablet to take notes. This might be a good idea for you if you have messy handwriting or you are simply more comfortable typing than you are writing. Just be sure to completely charge your device before class and save your notes multiple times during the class. Keep backups of your notes online or with a portable hard drive.

Evernote is a popular app that you can download to your tablet or laptop to keep your notes organized. It's like a digital notebook where you can create "notebooks" that can be labeled by class, and individual notes can be labeled by subject and date. Evernote offers both a free and premium version, but the free version is likely sufficient for you to take class notes.

Alternatives to Evernote are Word documents organized in folders or basic note apps.

The Old-Fashioned Way

Notebooks and pencils are still a good standby for notetaking. Purchase a separate notebook for each class or purchase a large binder and use dividers to separate your notes for each class. For a modern touch, you can use bullet journals to make your notes more visually appealing and fun to look at. You can learn more about bullet journaling by reading The Bullet Journal Method by Ryder Carroll, or you can Google bullet journals for notetaking and find a wealth of information on this topic.

Four Notetaking Tips

1.   Only write down the most important points.
Do not make the mistake of trying to write down every word that your professor says. You won't be able to do it, and you will miss something important in the process. Good notes should be simple and concise.
For example, if your instructor says, "Good morning students. Today we are going to talk about the anatomy of the heart. The human heart has 4 chambers..."
The only thing you need to write is this: heart has 4 chambers. It's simple and to the point.
2.   Sit where you can easily see.
Regardless of where your friends sit, you need to be in the front of the class if you have any type of vision problems or issues seeing the front of the class. Sitting in the front will also make it easier for you to pay attention.
3.   Put dates and headings on your notes.
You are going to take a ton of notes for every class, so it's important to clearly label them so that you can easily find what you are looking for when it's time to study. Record the date and the exam that this subject will show up on at the top of the page. This will make it much easier to assemble only the notes that you need to focus on for each exam.
4.   Review your notes with a highlighter after class.
It's a good idea to spend at least 15-30 minutes reviewing your notes after class or before you go to sleep at night (do both if you can). Studies show that reviewing your notes within 24 hours helps it stick with you longer. Some students even choose to rewrite their notes.

Use a highlighter to mark anything that your instructor seemed to emphasize during the lecture or anything that you want to spend extra time studying later.

Know Your Learning Style and Use It

You probably already know your learning style, but here is a quick overview of the three major learning styles: visual, auditory, and kinesthetic, in case you've never considered it an idea on how to study according to your personal style. Other learning styles are verbal, logical, social, and solitary. This short section should help you get some good ideas to help you start thinking about ways that you study best. I have included a section of books and websites on learning styles in the back of this book that will help you dive into this subject further. Your learning center can also be a helpful resource to help you discover how you learn best.

Don't be afraid to experiment with different methods of studying. If you are an auditory learner, don't waste hours staring at your textbook. If you're a kinesthetic learner, don't beat yourself up about not retaining information from lectures. You can find ways to master the material that fits better with your natural learning style. Some students learn best using a variety of methods from different learning styles, so don't be afraid to mix it up either.

1. The Visual Learner

Visual learners learn best by reading information written on the board, studying textbooks, watching videos, or seeing pictures and diagrams. You may enjoy doodling, taking notes, and making outlines in order to understand a concept better. Bullet journals are a popular way to make colorful notes and fancy drawings to reinforce what you are studying.

Look for visual aids that help you to understand what you are studying. Flashcards that include lots of images might be a good way to quiz yourself on the material before an exam.

2. The Auditory Learner

Auditory learners learn best through sound or music. They typically retain more from listening to a lecture or an audiobook than reading a book. You may want to record your lectures on your smartphone and listen to them again to reinforce the important concepts that your instructor presented in class.

You may also enjoy discussing a topic with a tutor or study group. Auditory learners often comprehend material better by reading aloud. Consider recording yourself reading the material and listen to your recording while you work out or cook dinner. You may also enjoy coming up with rhymes to help you remember material better if you are a musical person.

3. The Kinesthetic Learner

Kinesthetic learners need physical movement, touch, and hands-on activities to be at their best. Flashcards are an effective way to integrate movement and touch into your studies. You might also enjoy playing trivia games with your study group. Sometimes drawing pictures, doodling, and mind mapping will help you to understand concepts better. You might also read material better while standing or even walking on a treadmill (you'll get your workout in at the same time).
Take a look at the resources chapter at the back of this book to see recommended books, audiobooks, study guides, YouTube channels, and websites that you can use to help you learn according to your learning style.

Form a Study Group

The amount of material that you will be expected to know for exams can be overwhelming to tackle on your own. I strongly recommend that you join a study group of like-minded students or put one together yourself. The only reason that you should not join a study group is if you don't study well in groups. Some learners study better by themselves. If that's you, feel free to skip this section. I'll share an alternative to study groups in the next section that might work better for solitary learners.

Study groups offer the following benefits:

Accountability: When you know that your study partners are relying on you to do your part in the group, you are less likely to procrastinate on studying.

Support: Some groups plan regular activities to provide opportunities to talk and have fun together so that it's easier to keep study sessions all business. You can also save the last 30 minutes or so for chatting or downtime as a reward for staying on task.

Practice teamwork: Nurses need to know how to work well with others. Working with a study group is good practice in how to work closely with unique individuals for a common goal.

Gain unique perspectives on the material: Discussing the material with your study partners will allow you to see the material differently than you might have understood it while reading at home.

Tips on How to Have a Successful Study Group

Limit your group invites to only 3-6 very responsible students. Your study group will only be as successful as the students that you choose. This is not the time to invite your best friend who is barely passing and isn't interested in putting in the work necessary to do better. Target the brightest and most dedicated students in your classes. It's also important to consider the learning styles of everyone in the group and make sure that they are compatible. Discuss early on how you would like to study together.

Divide and teach the material to each other. One of the best ways to master the large amount of reading that you are expected to know is to divide the assignments between the members of your group. Each student will take detailed notes on their individual section of the reading and teach the most important details to the group. This only works well in small groups of very dedicated and responsible students. When everyone does their part, it works beautifully. Teaching the material to your study buddies will also reinforce the material in your own mind. Bonus!

Be organized and efficient with your study sessions. Agree on a regular study time and place so that everyone is on the same page. Stay consistent with your meeting times so there is no confusion about when and where you are meeting. You also need to agree ahead of time what you are going to focus on each session. If you plan to divide up the material, agree on this well in advance so that everyone has enough time to prepare.

Limit your study time to 2-3 hours and take breaks. Remember what you learned about the Pomodoro Technique; short focused blocks of time are more effective than hours of studying with no breaks. Just be sure to get back on task quickly after your break. Consider using a timer on your phone to signal when it's time to get back to work. After about 4 hours, everyone will start to lose focus, so have a set stopping time and stick to it.

Quiz each other on the material. Take practice tests with your study group or make up your own mini quizzes to help one another learn. Trivia nights and flashcard games are other fun ways to gain a better grasp of the material and enjoy the process. Who says studying has to be boring?

Rotate bringing healthy snacks and drinks. Studying is always better with good food. Challenge your study partners to bring healthy snacks that will provide energy rather than sugary snacks that will cause you all to crash by the end of the session. Vegetables and hummus, popcorn, fruit salad, and mixed nuts are just a few ideas. Don't forget to stay hydrated too. Water is a much better choice over soda and juices that are full of sugar.

Use Social Media to Excel in Your Classes

You might be surprised to know that Facebook can be used as a tool to help you in your classwork if you use it wisely. There are several large Facebook groups that you can join to help you stay on top of the most important news in the world of nursing and search for jobs from all over the world. Check out the Resources for Your Journey section at the back of the book for a list of the groups that I recommend.

Another way to use Facebook groups, that will save you time and help you stay organized is to create a private Facebook group for you and a select group of classmates or your study group. Use this group to communicate about assignment due dates, ask questions about things you didn't understand in your reading assignments, and share tips and study guides (I'll show you how to make your own study guides in the next section). Use Dropbox or Google Drive to share large documents like study guides within your group. If you are using this group to communicate with your study group, you can share a live calendar to keep track of study sessions and responsibilities.

The private chat feature allows you to vent your frustrations about your classes or instructors. If the thought of forming a study group makes you cringe, and you enjoy studying alone, a Facebook group might be the perfect tool for you to gain some of the benefits of a study group without having to step too far out of your comfort zone.

How to Create a Facebook Group
It's very easy to create a Facebook group and it's completely free:
1.   Sign into your personal Facebook account.
2.   On your Newsfeed page, click on "Groups" under the Explore menu on the left.
3.   Click the "Create Group" button on the top right of the screen.
4.   Complete the group settings page by entering a group name, selecting your privacy settings, and inviting your classmates.
Make sure that you start a closed group by invite only so that members feel safe to vent about classes.

Create Your Own Study Guides
The Pareto Principle states that 80% of your results will typically come from 20% of your effort or output (Richard Koch, *The 80/20 Principle: The Secret to Achieving More with Less* 1999). This means that when you find out what study strategies are most effective for your personal learning style, you can zero in on those strategies to have the most success. It also means that you can find the most important information that you need to know for a test in about 20% of the reading material. So how do you figure out what that 20% is and master that material in order to ace your exams?

Making your own study guides is an effective way to learn and commit the most important concepts to memory because you can focus in on creating questions based on the key concepts of each chapter only, and then test your knowledge until you have them committed to memory. It might sound like a lot of work, but the process is fairly simple, and the process of making the study guides alone will help you to grasp the material.

You can create study guides on your own or in a study group and share your guide with your study buddies.

Tips to Make Your Own Study Guides:
1)   Search for the 20% of the information that you need to know in your reading assignment. Textbooks typically make it pretty easy to see what the key concepts are. Zero in on concepts that your instructor emphasized in class.

2)   Create questions that will help you recall the most important information. You don't need to spend a lot of time making questions that are worthy of being placed on the NCLEX exam. As long as your questions help you to understand the information and recall it during your studies, they are good questions.

3)   Print several copies of your study guide and practice answering your questions. The first time you use your study guide, allow yourself to use your book when you need it. When you are done, check over your work using your book to ensure that you answered each question with complete accuracy.

4)   Study the areas that you were weakest at and try again. Go back and study the material that you had difficulty recalling and then take your practice exam again. When you are ready, challenge yourself to take the exam without using your book and see how many questions you get right. Do this as many

times as you need to recall all of the information without looking it up.

While this method sounds very simple, it works wonders. Learning to extract the most important information from any text is an important skill that will help you learn anything in life. You can use this to help you ace your NCLEX in conjunction with a good study guide. Give it a try and share this method with your classmates.

More Tips to Avoid Distractions
In addition to spending focused attention to your tasks for short intervals of time, you can try these simple techniques to cut out all distractions.

Be Prepared Before You Sit Down to Study or Work on a Project
Take care of any physical needs like going to the restroom or grabbing something to eat or drink before you sit down to study. Know exactly what you need to get done and gather all of your needed materials before you get started.

You can also mentally prepare for studying by writing down any pressing things that may need your attention. By writing them down, you are telling yourself that you will attend to this matter later and that it's okay to devote your full attention to studying now.

Turn off the TV, Music, Audiobooks, and Talk Radio
While many people think that they study better with background noise like music or the sound of the TV, several studies have shown that background noises can be more distracting than we realize. Your brain needs to work harder to decipher between what you are trying to focus on and the other noises that it is processing.

Put Your Cellphone Away While You Are Studying

There is nothing more distracting than seeing a notification pop up on your phone while you're trying to focus on a task. Do yourself a favor and turn it off or at least put it on the silent mode and out of your line of sight while you are studying. Trust me, the world will not end if you don't check those notifications for 25 minutes.

Avoid the Internet

Unless you are doing research, stay off the internet and turn off your email notifications. Checking your social media accounts for "only five minutes" before you start studying is an easy way to get to a late start. Instead, make checking your email or social media account your reward for completing your tasks.

Diffuse Essential Oils to Improve Concentration

Lavender, rosemary, and peppermint oils have been shown to increase concentration and memory retention. Dab a little on your wrists or diffuse the oils in the room that you are studying in.

Tutor Assistance

Tutor assistance is a matter that needs to be addressed at the start of the semester. Many nursing students wait until they've struggled through three or four tests to secure a good tutor, and they are often out of luck. Don't wait until it's too late to at least explore what your program offers so that you know what's available to you when you need some extra help.

I had a stroke years ago and I knew immediately something didn't feel right. I would read and read and wouldn't be able to recollect the content. It was more like my memory wasn't synchronizing. I'm a visual learner, so I would sometimes read chapters two or three times and still, it would not stick. I had a tutor who showed me a different way of remembering things, and I would use all sorts of techniques to jog my memory. I was very grateful for the tutors who had patience with me and showed me memory tricks to help me recall the information to do well on my exams.

Again, don't wait until you need extra help to find out what type of assistance is available to you in your program. Never be too prideful to ask for help. This is your future, and you need to do everything you can to ensure that you are successful so that you can become the best nurse that you can be.

Discipline and Train Your Mind

"Your mind is working at its best when you're being paranoid. You explore every avenue and possibility of your situation at high speed with total clarity." Banksy.

I don't know if you've noticed, but your mind controls your body. A good example is when you feel too tired to read, and then you see some of your classmates heading for the library to prepare for a test and Bam! You just feel the adrenaline rushing through your body and you get inspired and join them; this is the power of the mind. Conversely, if you have a negative attitude towards the reading assignment that is due tomorrow, you're going to have a difficult time sitting through it, even if you're full of energy.

Successful students train their mind with positive and empowering thoughts. Our brains are like the rest of our bodies. When you eat high-quality, healthy foods, your body will perform at an optimum level. When you fill your minds with motivating and inspiring thoughts, you can accomplish everything you set out to do. I've had loads of nursing school tests in my life, and I can tell you that you won't pass unless you discipline your mind and have a positive mindset.

Here are a few simple ways to build a positive mindset:

Recognize your go-to negative thoughts: We all have default negative thoughts such as, "things always go wrong for me," or "I'm not smart enough," or "I could never do that." It's important to recognize the negative thoughts that you experience on a regular basis and replace them with more empowering thoughts. For example, if I know that I often think, "I'm not smart enough," every time I have that thought from now on, I will make a conscious effort to remind myself: "I am just as smart as the top student in my class, and I have everything that it takes to become an excellent nurse." Yes, it will take a lot of effort, and the change won't happen overnight, but over time you can start to change your default thinking and become a more positive person.

Surround yourself with positive quotes and inspiring thoughts. Place sticky notes or index cards all over your home with quotes that keep you going. Write your favorite quotes in your notebook or student planner where you'll see them every time you study.

Listen to motivational videos and audiobooks to help you reframe your mindset. There are a ton of motivational videos online that you can listen to for free. If you are new to the world of motivational speakers, try listening to people like Tony Robbins, Lisa Nichols, John Maxwell, Dale Carnegie, Eric E.T. Thomas, or Mel Robbins. As you listen, write down the nuggets of wisdom that you would like to remember and review them daily until you start seeing a change.

Spend time with positive people. If you hang around positive (or negative people) long enough, they will rub off on you. Be wise about the people that you surround yourself with. Positivity is a two-way street. Do your best to stay positive and motivate your friends and they will be more likely to reciprocate.

Tips to Improve Your Memory and Brain Function

You've probably heard that some neuroscientists believe that the average person only uses about ten percent of their brain. Over the last decade, science has learned a lot more about what the brain is capable of and how we can play a part in helping our brain to function better. How would you like to improve your memory and concentration by implementing a few simple daily habits?

Author, speaker, and "brain coach" Jim Kwik goes all over the world teaching entrepreneurs, athletes, celebrities, and students how to think smarter and faster, make confident decisions, read and recall information faster, and train their brains for optimal performance. Here are five tips that he teaches people to do first thing in the morning to improve overall brain function.

Five Simple Habits to Improve Your Memory and Brain Function

1.   Make your bed as soon as you get out of it.
I know that this sounds too simple but making your bed right when you get up (even before you check your phone) gives you a small mental win that sets you up for excellence the rest of the day. According to Jim, "how you do anything is how you do everything." So, starting your day by doing something productive, you are already training your brain to keep commitments to yourself and follow your routine. It's also nice to come home to a neatly made bed at the end of the day.

Try it for a month and watch the difference it makes in your day.

2.   Drink 16 ounces of water.

Forming new habits can be hard to do, so I recommend stacking habits after something you would normally do. Right after you wake up, make your bed, and then go straight to the kitchen and drink at least 16 ounces of water. Our bodies are made up of 75% water, so being dehydrated can seriously alter our brain function. Many studies have shown that people who are well-hydrated perform better on tests. We all wake up dehydrated, so it's vitally important to drink water first thing in the morning. If you are not used to drinking a lot of water, this might be difficult at first, but I suggest just standing there until you're able to drink it all. It will get easier over time.

Start your day with water and carry around a water bottle with you throughout the day.

3.   Take a cold shower

This simple tip is probably the most difficult (and strange) out of the five, but many people can attest to how cold-water therapy can improve your energy, brain function, and ability to fight disease. Jim recommends turning on the cold water in your shower for the last minute and allowing the cold water to hit your face and chest. According to Jim, it will be horrible for the first few days, and you may have to build up to a whole minute by adding on a few more seconds every day. Your body will get used to it after a few days and you will start to enjoy how your body feels after the cold shower.

4.   Brush your teeth with your opposite hand.

I found it fascinating to learn that we can improve our neural connections in our brains and even grow new ones — similar to the way we improve the way our body functions and grow larger muscles through exercise — by brushing our teeth with our opposite hand. If you write with your right hand, brush your teeth with your left hand for better brain health!

5.   Drink tea and journal.

Jim recommends making a tea of gotu kola, ginkgo, lion's mane, and MCT oil. All of these ingredients boost brain function and improve focus. Then he'll sit down with a journal and write as he sips on his tea. Jim points out that many geniuses such as Albert Einstein, Leonardo DaVinci, and Thomas Edison wrote in journals, and he suspects that journaling may have been part of why they were considered geniuses. He credits his journaling time with many of his most creative and profitable ideas.

Brain Food

Jim also recommends including plenty of foods that are rich in antioxidants, good fats, vitamins, and minerals. His top ten "brain foods" are the following:

1.   Avocado: good fat
2.   Blueberries (Jim calls brain berries): protects the brain and improves brain function
3.   Broccoli: rich in vitamin K which improves cognitive function
4.   Coconut oil: good fat
5.   Eggs: contains choline which improves memory; a good source of vitamin E
6.   Green leafy vegetables (like spinach or kale): good source of vitamin E and folate
7.   Salmon and Sardines: source of DHA and omega-3s
8.   Turmeric: improves the brain's oxygen intake and keeps the immune system healthy
9.   Walnuts: high in antioxidants and magnesium
10.   Dark Chocolate (the darker the better): Improves focus and concentration

Do your best to add a few of these ingredients to your diet every day to improve your brain power. Jim recommends making a brain smoothie by blending together water, green leafy vegetables, blueberries, avocados, and coconut oil.

(Jim Kwik, "10 Morning Habits Geniuses Use to Jump Start the Brain for Maximum Learning & Productivity" Mindvalley, 2018)

Chapter Summary and Putting it into Action

Summary
Pomodoro Technique: A simple, yet powerful way to maximize your study time, stay focused, and make studying more enjoyable.
1)   Break down one larger task into smaller task that you can get done in short, 25-minute intervals.
2)   Set your timer for 25 minutes and focus your complete attention on one task until the timer goes off.
3)   Take a 5-minute break from your task. Get up and walk around.
4)   Start your timer again for another 25-minute pomodoro. Take a 15-to 30-minute break after every 3 or 4 pomodoros.

Notetaking Tips
Use the method that works best for you: laptop, tablet, bullet journal, or old-fashioned notebook.
1.   Only write down the most important points.
2.   Sit where you can easily see.
3.   Put dates and headings on your notes so that you can easily reference relevant notes for each exam.
4.   Review your notes with a highlighter after class. Mark anything that your instructor seemed to emphasize during the lecture or anything that you want to spend extra time studying later.

Know Your Learning Style

Consider what ways you learn best and experiment with different study methods that fit your learning style.

Visual Learners: Learn best by reading textbooks, watching videos, looking at images or charts.
Some ideas to study for visual learners:
- Make outlines
- Bullet Journal
- Draw charts and diagrams
- Create flashcards with images

Auditory Learners: Learn best through sound or music. They often learn more from listening to lectures than reading textbooks.
Some ideas to study for auditory learners:
- Record your lectures and listen to them later
- Read out loud and record yourself reading
- Discuss the material with a study partner or tutor
- Come up with rhymes to help you remember important material

Kinesthetic Learner: Learns best through physical movement, touch, and hands-on activities.
Some ideas to study for kinesthetic learners:
- Flashcards to get your hands involved
- Trivia games
- Draw pictures of the material
- Mind mapping
- Read while standing up or walking on a treadmill

Benefits of a Study Group
- Accountability: When you know that your study partners are relying on you to do your part in the group, you are less likely to procrastinate on studying.
- Support: Some groups plan regular activities to provide opportunities to talk and have fun.
- Practice teamwork: Nurses need to know how to work well with others.
- Gain unique perspectives on the material

Use Facebook Groups to Excel
Organize a Facebook group to communicate with your classmates about assignments, share study guides, and vent about your frustrations.

Tips to Avoid Distractions

Be prepared before you sit down to study or work on a project. Take care of physical needs and get something to eat and drink. Gather all of your materials before you sit down to study.
Turn off the TV, music, audiobooks, and talk radio.
Put your cellphone away while you are studying. Do yourself a favor and turn it off or at least put it on silent and out of your line of sight while you are studying.
Avoid the internet. Unless you are doing research, stay off the internet and turn off your email notifications.
Include lots of the top ten "brain foods" in your diet:
1.   Avocado: good fat
2.   Blueberries (Jim calls brain berries): protects the brain and improves brain function
3.   Broccoli: rich in vitamin K which improves cognitive function
4.   Coconut oil: good fat
5.   Eggs: contains choline which improves memory; and a good source of vitamin E
6.   Green leafy vegetables (like spinach or kale): good source of vitamin E and folate
7.   Salmon and Sardines: source of DHA and omega-3s
8.   Turmeric: improves brain's oxygen intake and keeps the immune system healthy
9.   Walnuts: high in antioxidants and magnesium
10.   Dark Chocolate (the darker the better): Improves focus and concentration

Put it into Action
How to Form a Study Group

- Limit your group invites to only 3-6 very responsible students.
- Divide and teach the material to each other.
- Be organized and efficient with your study sessions. Agree on a regular study time and place so that everyone is on the same page. Stay consistent.
- Limit your study time to 2-3 hours and take breaks.
- Quiz each other on the material. Take practice tests with your study group
- Rotate bringing healthy snacks and drinks. Studying is always better with good food.

How to Create Your Own Study Guides
1) Search for the 20% of the information that you need to know in your reading assignment.
2) Create questions that will help you recall the most important information.
3) Print several copies of your study guide and practice answering your questions. The first time you use your study guide, allow yourself to use your book when you need it.
4) Study the areas that you were weakest at and try again.

Tutor Assistance
Visit your program's learning center to learn more about the programs and materials that are available to you.

Tips to Build a Positive Mindset: Successful students train their mind with positive and empowering thoughts.
• Recognize your go-to negative thoughts and replace them with more empowering thoughts.
• Surround yourself with positive quotes and inspiring thoughts.
• Listen to motivational videos and audiobooks to help you reframe your mindset.
• Spend time with positive people.

Five Simple Habits to Improve Your Memory and Brain Function

1.   Make your bed as soon as you get out of it. It gives you a small win first thing in the morning.

2.   Drink 16 ounces of water first thing in the morning.

3.   Take a cold shower to improve energy and brain function.

4.   Brush your teeth with your opposite hand. It improves the neural connections in your brain.

5.   Drink tea and journal.

Notes

Chapter Six

Simple Keys to Success

"Being a nurse isn't about grades, it's about being who we are. No book can teach you how to cry with a patient. No class can teach you how to tell their family that their parents have died or are dying. No professor can teach you how to find dignity in giving someone a bed bath. A nurse is not about the pills or charting. It's about being able to love people when they are at their weakest moments." Anonymous

Set goals and read them daily. "No one is ready for a thing until he believes he can acquire it. The state of mind must be belief, not mere hope or wish." — Napoleon Hill

Study after study shows that people who set specific, measurable goals are much more likely to achieve what they want out of life. I suggest that you set some goals for your nursing program beyond just receiving your degree and finding a job. Create a vision for yourself of the kind of student you will be and the job that you will receive after you graduate. Consider the following questions to get you started:

What kind of grades do you want to get?
How many hours should you study per week to get the grades you want?
What will your GPA be at graduation?

Is there a certain program you want to be part of?

What will your specialty be?

Where do you want to work when you graduate?

Once you've decided on a goal or two, write them down and post your goal somewhere you will see it every day like your bathroom mirror or your fridge. You should review your goals at least two times every day to keep them at the forefront of your mind. When you do this, your brain will begin looking for ways to make your goals happen. Write out a plan to achieve each goal and schedule the action steps in your weekly schedule.

Treat teachers as coaches.

Your teachers are there to help you become the best nurse that you can be. Treat each one like a superstar coach who can share their years of experience and help you to avoid mistakes that they might have made in their career. Ask questions and soak up all of the knowledge you can in every class. You can learn something from every teacher, even your least favorite teacher. See Chapter 8 for details on how to deal with difficult instructors and why it's important to establish a relationship with them early in the year.

Start a study group with the smartest students in your class.

No matter how dedicated or intelligent you are, there is always going to be someone smarter than you in every class. This is great news! Once you discover who this person is, ask them to join your new study group. Challenge yourself to study hard and contribute to your super-smart classmate so that they feel compelled to help you out too. Top students understand that they can always learn from others and they want to be around those who stretch them to be at their best. Better yet, recruit the top 2 or 3 students in your classes and form a super team!

Take advantage of learning centers.

A learning center provides students with the materials, tools, and instruction to understand concepts that they might not have understood in class. Even if you are acing every one of your exams, you should visit the learning center on your campus and see what they have to offer. You may find that you need a little extra help in a subject down the line, and you'll feel much more comfortable coming in when you are struggling if you are already familiar with what is available to you. At the very least, your learning center may have valuable books that you can borrow or read on site to help you prepare for your exams.

Learning centers are also important for any student dealing with a learning disability like dyslexia or ADHD. You may be able to receive a personalized learning plan that will help you master the concepts that you need to know to succeed in your program.

Immerse yourself in your craft.
One of the best ways to stay motivated and constantly growing in your field is to immerse yourself in your craft. You can do this by listening to podcasts, watching YouTube videos, reading blogs, listening to audiobooks, and joining social media groups for nurses, etc.

Choose a method of immersion that is enjoyable to you and makes sense with your lifestyle. If you hate social media, don't waste your time joining Facebook groups for nurses. If you love watching videos on your phone, subscribe to a few good YouTube channels made for nurses. If you like to listen to something while you work out, try a nursing podcast or audiobook. By choosing something you enjoy, you'll have a better chance of following through long term.

The final chapter of this book is full of recommended resources and tools to help you become the best nurse you can be.

Prioritize self-care

I know that I've already mentioned this a few times in this book, but it's just as important to take care of yourself as it is to study and go to class. If you don't take time to eat right, exercise, get good quality sleep, and decompress daily, you cannot operate at your best. Pulling too many all-nighters, eating a junk food diet, and not exercising is a recipe to make yourself sick, burned out, and unfocused.

Take care of yourself. Your body and brain will thank you. And forming habits of self-care will make it easier for you to maintain them long after graduation.

Chapter Summary and Putting it into Action

Summary

Simple Keys to Success

1. Write down your goals.
2. Treat teachers as coaches.
3. Start a study group with someone smarter than you.
4. Take advantage of learning centers.
5. Immerse yourself in your craft.
6. Prioritize self-care.

Put it into Action

1. Write down your goals.
- Set goals beyond just passing your classes.
- Post them where you can see them daily.
- Read them to yourself at least twice per day.

2. Treat teachers as coaches.
- Soak up their experience.
- Meet with tough teachers early in the year and ask questions.
- You may need references from your teachers later in the year, so make a good impression.

3.   Start a study group with the smartest students in your classes.

•   Look for the smartest person in your class and ask to start a study group with them.

•   This will challenge you to be the best you can be.

•   Do your best to challenge them to be better and they will return the favor.

4.   Take advantage of learning centers.

•   Visit the learning center early in the year so you know what is offered.

•   If you have a learning disability, this is a great place to get customized help.

•   Learning centers are an important resource for every student.

5.   Immerse yourself in your craft.

•   Smart students and nurses are constantly learning and growing in their craft.

•   Choose a format that you enjoy: blogs, audiobooks, YouTube videos, social media, etc.

•   Check out the resources chapter at the back of this book for recommendations.

6.   Prioritize self-care.

•   If you want to be a successful student, you need to eat right, exercise, get good quality sleep, and take time to decompress every day

Notes

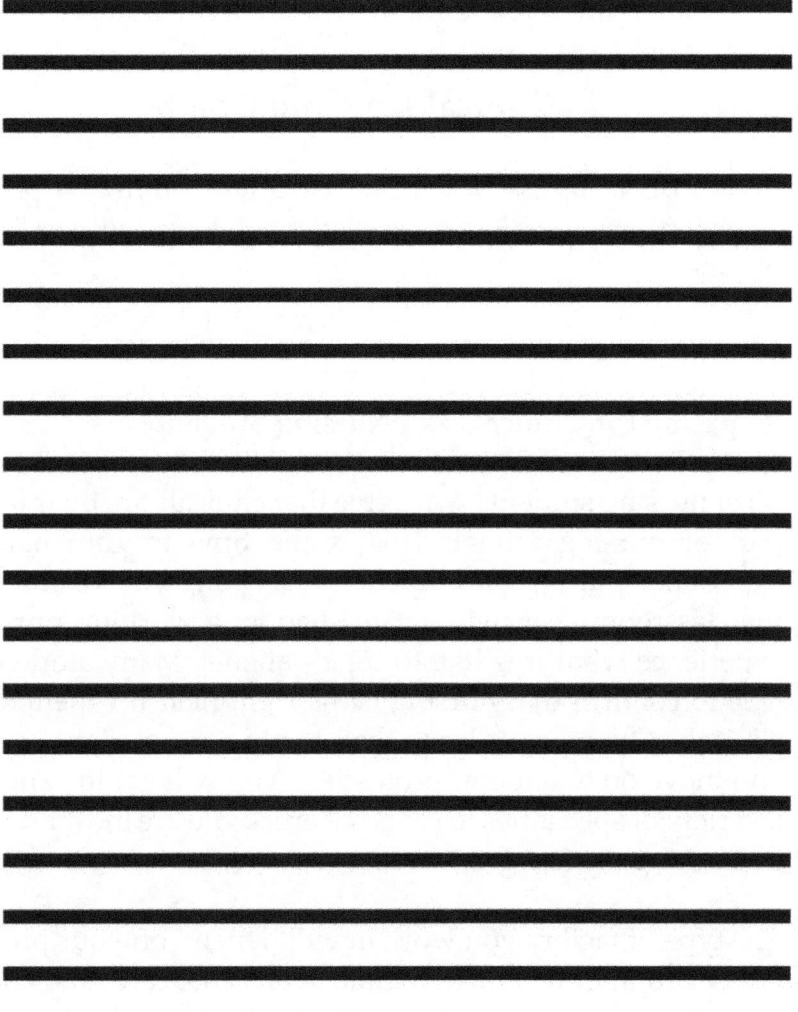

Chapter Seven

Clinical Do's and Don'ts

"You treat a disease, you win, you lose. You treat a person, I guarantee you, you'll win, no matter what the outcome." Patch Adams

Preparing for Clinicals as a Nursing Student

Most nursing students will agree that clinicals are their favorite part of nursing school. This is the time to gain hands-on experience putting into practice everything you've studied in the classroom. You will get to shadow a working nurse and experience what it is like to treat patients. Many students are able to confirm that nursing is the right field for them during clinicals. Others may learn that nursing is not right for them and move on to another profession. You will get to experience a variety of specialties to see what areas you are most interested in working in after graduation.

The type of facility you work in will depend on your program. Every program will include time in an acute care hospital. You may also have rotations in public health, mental health centers, and outpatient facilities. Shift times and durations will also vary based on your program. Typically, you will be scheduled for 8 or 12-hour shifts. Once you complete a shift, you will be scheduled for your next shift.

It is normal to be nervous when you are starting your first clinical rotations. Every day will bring new experiences, pressures, and challenges. Just remember that every nurse has gone through the same process as you and survived. Clinicals are designed to prepare you for real-life experiences that you will encounter after you become a licensed nurse, so embrace this learning opportunity for what it is, and don't put any extra pressure on yourself.

Clinical Do's and Don'ts for Success

Do Get There Early
You want to get there early so that you can choose the best patients for you. Review the patient's chart and make sure that you understand their condition. If you don't, you shouldn't be treating that patient. Some students think it's important to choose the most challenging cases to prove themselves. While this might sound good in theory, it's important to make sure that you don't get in over your head. Remember that you are dealing with real lives.

Showing up early also shows your instructors and everyone you will be working with on your shift that you are a professional and that you care about your work and education.

Don't Forget Your Supplies
Before you start your first clinical rotation, you need to verify which supplies you'll need to bring in your clinical bag and which supplies will be provided for you. Get into the habit of double checking that you have all of your necessary equipment packed in your clinical bag long before each shift starts. There is nothing worse than being late because you are running around your house trying to find something you need at the last minute.

Do Put in Extra Study Time

In order to be successful in clinicals, you have got to put in the study time. It's not only about the time that you spend studying to pass your exams. Spend some extra time studying the things that will help you do your best in your clinicals. You won't be expected to know everything, but you should take some time to prepare for each specialty rotation. If you are working in a pediatric rotation, focus on common pediatric diagnoses and treatments.

Once you are assigned a patient, take the time to prepare by getting organized, taking detailed notes, and making sure that you understand everything about your patient's condition, medications, procedures, and treatment plan. If you have questions, it's better to ask than guess. Mistakes can put your patient's life at stake. When in doubt, always ask.

Don't Get Involved in the Drama

Every workplace has its share of drama, bullies, and gossip. Avoid it all and remember why you are there. Drama will steal your focus and bring negativity that you don't need in your life. You are there to make a better life for yourself and your family and learn how to make a difference in the lives of your patients. Stay focused on your goals, and don't allow anyone to get you off track.

Sexual harassment and racial or gender discrimination are serious issues that you should never tolerate in any workplace, including clinical shifts. Speak to your instructor or school administrator right away. Not only should you stand up for yourself so that the harassment or discrimination will stop, but you might prevent future students from being subjected to the same horrible situation. You have a legal right to a safe workplace. Read Chapter 8 for more information on these important topics.

Do Care About Your Patients More Than Protocol

Nursing students can sometimes get so focused on doing everything exactly right that they forget that they are treating an actual person. While it is vital to focus on following protocols to treat your patients in the best manner possible, part of being a great nurse is showing compassion, giving a warm smile, and making your patient as comfortable as possible.

When you first meet your patient, introduce yourself and ask permission to be their student nurse. Do your best to make your patient feel comfortable with you. Treat him or her as a person and not just a case study. Your patients can tell when you honestly care about their well-being.

Don't Expect Perfection

Clinicals will give you a taste of the unpredictability of the life of a working nurse. You will work with all kinds of patients with unique personalities and backgrounds. There will be coworkers that annoy you and others that you'll want to stay in touch with after you graduate. Some days will be fulfilling and fun. On other days, you'll feel like you can't do anything right, and you'll want to quit. Just remember that every nurse has bad days. Do your best to stay positive and make the best of each day.

Do Make Friends

Nursing is all about working as a team of professionals to provide the best possible care for your patients. Registered nurses work with other RNs, LPNs, CNAs, and other professionals every day. Help out your fellow nursing students when you can because you never know when you will need their help. Be as helpful as possible to those you are shadowing, and they will be excited to teach you all of their inside secrets.

Don't Waste a Day

There is so much for you to learn in clinicals. Soak up all of the knowledge you can every day. Ask questions, take notes, and make the most of every shift. If you don't understand something, ask. There is no way for you to learn everything that you need to know before you get there, so get comfortable learning on the job. If you struggled in a certain area, make a note to review that subject during your study time. Don't just do enough to get by; make the most of this time.

Do Ask and Answer Questions

Clinicals are not the time to fake it until you make it. Remember that this time is tailor-made for you to learn. Ask lots of questions and take good notes. If your instructor asks questions about a procedure or medical condition, take the opportunity to show that you know your stuff. Just like the classroom, you will get out of clinicals as much as you put into it.

Don't Avoid Procedures

If you are assigned to perform a procedure, don't try to get out of it. Ask questions when you need help, but don't ever back down from the challenge. The only way that you can become an excellent nurse is to gain this hands-on experience, so make the most of it. If you make a mistake, remember that every nurse makes mistakes, and learn from it so that you don't make the same mistake twice.

Do Enjoy the Ride

Clinicals can be a lot of fun. You've studied hard to get to this point, and now you get to actually do the hands-on work. Allow yourself to enjoy the experience. Get to know the people that you work with, as well as your patients. Be intentional about doing everything you can to make the lives of your patients better while they are with you.

Smile, laugh, and enjoy the ride. It will be over before you know it!

A Note About Nursing Diagnosis

One thing that is important to remember is that you are becoming a nurse, not a doctor, so you need a nursing diagnosis, not a medical doctor diagnosis. So, you're going to make diagnoses that could be caused by the main diagnosis or a symptom that it's related to.

For example, nowadays, many people aren't sleeping, so insomnia is a huge one. "Disturbed sleep pattern" would be a nurse's diagnosis. "Insomnia" would be the diagnosis from the doctor. Make sure that you understand the difference so that you are making the correct diagnosis and creating the proper care plan for your patients.

Chapter Summary and Putting it into Action

Summary

Clinicals will provide you with hands-on experience to practice what you've learned in the classroom. Prepare for your shifts and stay organized so that you can provide the best possible care for your patients. You will not be expected to know everything, so don't be afraid to ask questions.

DO:

☐   Get there early and bring your supplies: Get into the habit of making sure that you have all of your supplies in your bag long before your shift starts.

☐   Put in extra study time: Review the common diagnosis and procedures for the specialty that you are working in.

☐   Care about your patients more than protocol: Your patients want to feel like human beings and not just another case study.

☐   Make friends: Nursing is about working together as a team.

☐   Ask and answer questions: Remember that you are there to learn so never be afraid to ask questions. Answer questions whenever you can to show that you know your stuff.

☐   Enjoy the ride: Stay positive and allow yourself to enjoy your work.

Bonus tip: Know the difference between a nursing diagnosis and a medical doctor diagnosis.

DON'T:

☐   Get involved in the drama: Drama, complaining, and gossip can create a negative environment and distract you from your purpose. Avoid it!

☐   Expect perfection: There will be rough days. Try to stay positive and make the best of each shift.

☐   Waste a day: If you struggled in a certain area, make a note to review that subject during your study time. Don't just do enough to get by; make the most of this time.

☐   Avoid procedures: If you are assigned to perform a procedure, don't try to get out of it. Ask questions when you need help, but don't ever back down from the challenge.

Notes

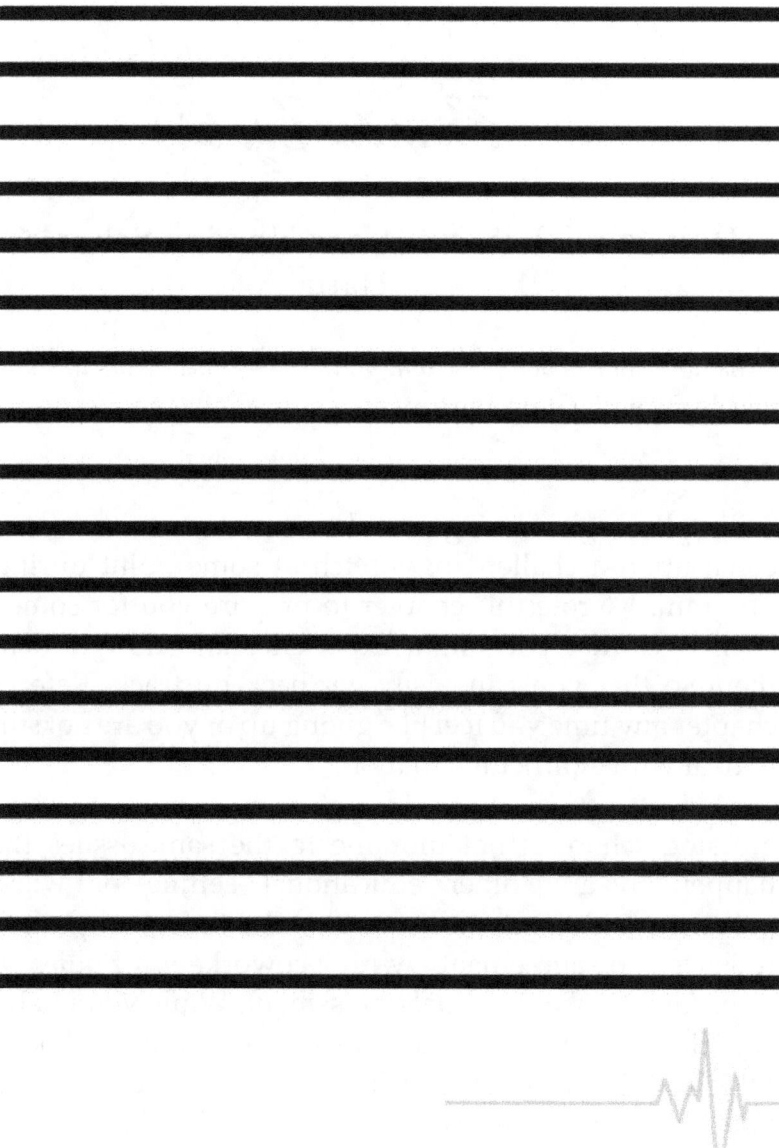

Chapter Eight

How to Stick it Out When Nursing School Gets Hard

"The door that nobody else will go in at, seems always to swing open widely for me." Clara Barton

Sailing through nursing school does not mean that you won't come upon a challenging stretch at some point during your program. I wrote this chapter to prepare you for some of the challenges that you might experience and how to deal with them so that you can easily get back on track. Refer to this chapter any time you feel like giving up or you are not sure how to deal with a difficult situation.

Nursing school is not immune to the same issues that can happen in any other educational setting or workplace: problems with instructors, long work hours, bad performance reviews, disagreement with coworkers, bullies, racial discrimination, and sexual harassment. While you likely won't experience all of these situations in your nursing school career, I think it's important to touch on a few of these issues and give you some tools to deal with them in case they happen to you or one of your coworkers.

If you take nothing else away from this chapter, I want you to know that any type of harassment or discrimination is illegal, and you have the right to stand up for yourself and demand it to stop.

Dealing with Instructor Problems

I have completed my LVN, ADN, BSN, and MSN program, and now I am working on my master's degree in nursing, so I can tell you that I have experienced many levels of nursing school. In my experience, there is always at least one difficult instructor in every program. Even when you do your best, there is usually that one professor who seems to be recalcitrant.

I was pregnant during my LVN program, and I was a little sensitive during the early part of my pregnancy, due to hormones. It was a 12-month program, which was a lot to handle for anyone, especially during pregnancy. During the first semester, professors are typically trying to wean you out of the program. I had one instructor that was so hard on me, that she even hit me one time in clinical when I was inserting a peripheral intravenous catheter in a patient, and she told me, "no, no, no..." My classmate, the patient, and I looked at her in astonishment. We could not believe that she did that. Of course, she didn't care; she had a rough personality.

When graduation came, she actually had the nerve to come behind me and put up bunny ears while I took a photo with my family. I was shocked. My mother and grandmother (who are both nurses) told me that I can learn from anyone and that she was only hard on me because she saw potential in me. I told my grandmother that I wished she didn't see potential in me, but I remembered this advice as she continued to stay on me throughout the year. I noticed that the students that she ignored didn't do so well and many of them did not go on to become nurses.

Although it was difficult to deal with this tough teacher, I survived, and she helped me become a better nurse. I am thankful for that. You too will survive your difficult instructors. Here are some tips on how to deal with them.

SET UP A MEETING: As a student nurse, you are becoming a professional soon, so you've got to act like one. Set up a meeting with the instructor to talk about what's bothering you and discuss his or her expectations of you. Often times you'll learn that this "tough instructor" really does have your best interests at heart and is willing to help you succeed. Don't waste half of the year being stressed about a difficult teacher; make an appointment as soon as possible.

REPORT THEM: If you are not able to resolve an issue with the instructor in a face-to-face meeting or you are dealing with an extremely sensitive issue like racial discrimination or sexual harassment, you need to file a report. You are paying good money to learn in a safe environment where your instructors should not in any way be a deterrent to your learning. If you know of other students who have similar complaints, ask them if they would be willing to file reports as well. Talk to the office of student affairs or whatever the equivalent is at your school and find out the process required to file a complaint.

BE CONFIDENT AND KIND: Don't allow the instructor to snatch your confidence from you; don't permit her to get the best of you. Always be courteous and professional with every professor. As a nurse, you will have to get used to dealing with coworkers, bosses, and patients with all kinds of personalities. Some will be difficult. Hang in there and remember that the semester won't last forever.

How to Make Your Toughest Teacher Your Biggest Ally

On the subject of difficult teachers, you will most likely have at least one instructor who will challenge you more than the rest during your program. I'm not talking about an instructor that you have a personal problem with. I'm talking about that instructor that every student complains about because their tests are so hard that no one can possibly pass them.

Meet with this teacher early in the year and bring a few questions with you. Most students will shy away from the tougher teachers, so this will make you stand out (which helps later on when you need references), and you will probably learn that this teacher is not too different from your other teachers. While other students might dread this teacher's class, you will go in there with a positive attitude that will take you much farther.

Jon Haws RN and creator of the popular podcast and blog NRSNG recommends that you meet with your toughest instructor right after your first exam and say the following:

"I feel like I studied really hard for this test, I read all the assigned reading (because you did), I took the practice tests, I felt like I understood the material in class . . . but my grade on this test has me a bit discouraged . . . I've always been a good student . . . what can I do to better prepare for your exams."

According to Jon, you will learn so much more than the other students who are too busy complaining about how difficult the exam was. You will gain insight into how this instructor writes their exams that will help you to do better the next time. The toughest instructors typically teach higher level classes so having a relationship with them can be a huge benefit. Nurse Haws says that he stays in touch with the toughest instructors that he had in school and has used them as references many times over the years. (Hawes, Jon. "How to Talk to Nursing Professors (even when they don't want to talk to you)" NRSNG Podcast. Podcast audio. March 2016)

Recognizing Intimidators at Work

Everywhere you find yourself working with human beings, do not forget that "to err is human…" You may get to an office and meet all the workers who appear calm and beaming, but do not always assume they are all cool with each other. It happens in almost every working environment. Workers in segmented offices may have less disputes in comparison to an open office, nursing, as well as nursing school is more of an open office environment. Bullies, gossip, discrimination, and harassment are unfortunately common issues.

Bullies

The American Nurses Association defines bullying as "repeated, unwanted harmful actions intended to humiliate, offend and cause distress in the recipient" (By Kathleen Colduvell, RN, BSN, BA, CBC, "Nurse Bullying: Stand Up and Speak Out" Nurse.org, 2015). I sincerely hope that you never experience bullying in your nursing program or in the workplace after you graduate. Unfortunately, bullying is common in our field.
One study conducted with Vanderbilt University Medical Center revealed that about 60% of new nurses leave their jobs within six months because of bullying.

If you think bullying only originates from instructors or those in a position of power, you are greatly mistaken. Unfortunately, bullying can occur between nursing students too. In the 80s, nursing professor Judith Meissner introduced the popular phrase, "nurses eat their young," and the phrase is still commonly used today. Some people choose not to like you for what seems like no good reason. They shout at you or threaten you for things that obviously don't matter. Many times, feelings of superiority are the reason bullying happens: when they feel they got through nursing school before you and probably have more experience than you do.

Bullying can prompt concerns about your wellbeing, unnecessary pressure, and a pointless distraction that can impair your ability to be efficient at work. Left unchecked, bullying can lead to larger problems like anger, depression, and leaving a position, so it's critical to learn ways to deal with intimidators in case you are faced with this unfortunate situation. Dealt with the right way, you can use this situation to develop personally and professionally.

So, when you encounter bullies in nursing school, how can you deal with them?

Don't Retaliate: It's not worth it. Retaliating may lead to violence and even getting kicked out of your program. If the authorities are called, they probably won't care about who started it. Be smart about how you handle the situation. Keep it professional at all times. This will not be the last difficult coworker that you have in your life, so take this as a learning opportunity.

Examine Yourself: Bullying is never your fault. No one has the right to treat you like you are less important than them or unworthy of your position in the program. However, it's always valuable to take a moment and consider whether you have played a role in this person's behavior towards you. Maybe it's some abandoned responsibility or attitude towards them that sparked the bully's ill-treatment of you. Recognizing your part in the situation (if any) may help you start a conversation and come to an understanding that ends the bullying.

Take Advantage of the Resources Available to You: Due to the fact that bullying has been a widespread problem within the nursing profession, many schools and medical facilities offer educational programs and materials on how to deal with bullying. Check with your learning center or school administration offices to see what is available to you.

Stand up to the Bully: Whether or not you have had a role to play in the mistreatment by a coworker, it's important to try to work things out with them before escalating the situation. Staying silent about the mistreatment is the equivalent of condoning it. Standing up to the bully shows the importance of keeping a civil and respectful environment for everyone.
You have the right to calmly, but firmly state that you will not tolerate this ill-treatment any longer.

Report the Bully: If you find it hard to walk up to the bullies and tell them they are not treating you well, talk to an instructor or an administrator. Many times, a bully will not admit to their behavior, so it is always a good idea to try and work things out with them first. You don't want to create a more difficult work environment for yourself by reporting a minor case of bullying, so use this as a last resort. If this person has a track record of bullying others, see if you can garner some support from the other victims.

Racial and Gender Discriminators
Discrimination is a major issue that no one should tolerate in any educational or work environment. According to the U.S. Equal Employment Opportunity Commission, "The law forbids discrimination when it comes to any aspect of employment, including hiring, firing, pay, job assignments, promotions, layoff, training, fringe benefits, and any other term

or condition of employment." If you ever find yourself the victim of discrimination of any kind, you have the legal right to speak up for yourself and expect it to stop.

Gender Bias and Discrimination
Studies show gender bias and even discrimination is common among men in nursing programs and in the workplace. One recent study showed that over 89% of men acknowledged anti-male comments made by instructors in the classroom (Men in Nursing, August 2006, Volume: 1 Number 4, page 43 – 49). Outcomes of gender bias are harmful to our profession and should not be tolerated. If you find yourself the victim of gender discrimination of any kind, regardless of your gender, you have the legal right to report it. Follow the tips at the end of this chapter to address the situation.

Dealing with Racism
When someone refuses to communicate with you at all for seemingly no good reason, you may be dealing with racism. If someone makes offensive comments regarding your race or ethnicity, you are certainly dealing with racial discrimination, and it is against the law.

I just recently went through a situation like this with my previous company. I had a manager who avoided me. She didn't want to communicate with me, she didn't want to show me anything, and for two years, I went through this racial discrimination. I even received pictures of a monkey and fried chicken from one of my managers. It was hard for me to report her simply because of her status, who she was in the area, and who her family was, but then when she started retaliating against me, I felt I had to finally stand up because it was getting out of hand. I went from supervising clinics five minutes from my home to driving forty-five minutes to a location to open up a clinic that I did not supervise.

Another way you could tell that a nursing supervisor, charge nurse, manager, or anybody is treating you unfairly is when you are on the medical floor and the charge nurse always gives you the highest acuity patients. That gives you a long night and a long day, and you end up going over 12 hours. That could be a sign of racial discrimination. You have to stand up for yourself in this situation.

Retribution
Retribution is a form of retaliation commonly carried out by the manager, instructor or any other person in a high-ranking position, but in nursing school, it is mostly from instructors. Retribution typically occurs for a reason that may or may not be fair. It could result from a past mistake or disrespect, and the outcome or punishment can come in many forms. It could be shift rescheduling, strict handling, colossal tasks, etc. Although there is a federal law against it, most of the time, the person responsible for it plays it smart and denies the charges. The only safe passage out of this is to report it to a higher authority, go up your chain of command, or if it is more than you think you can handle, then you have to report to the Equal Employment Opportunity Commission.

Tips to Deal with Bullying and Discrimination in the Workplace or School

Don't Wait Too Long to Say Something: The best time to address a bully or discriminator is as soon as you know for sure what is going on. At times, it may be difficult to tell whether an insensitive comment or action is simply the result of a bad day or something that needs to be addressed. However, if someone offends you, you have every right to speak up and let this person know that you will not tolerate it. As motivational speaker Lisa Nichols likes to say, "we teach people how to treat us."

Vent, But Don't Gossip: While you may need to vent your frustrations to another coworker, it's important to avoid starting gossip. If you need to vent, wait until after hours and talk over the phone or at another location to avoid having someone overhear your conversation. It's always best to address the offending party first before discussing the matter with others when possible.

Try to Stay Calm: Nurses are pros at acting cool under extreme pressure. Dealing with bullying or experiencing discrimination will test this ability. When addressing the situation with the offending party or an administrator, try to stay calm and simply state the facts.

Keep Track of the Details: If you think that you might need to report someone, keep careful notes about the offensive actions with dates, times, locations, etc. This information can be extremely helpful in the event that the offending party denies the details of your report.

Dominate the Stress: Bullying and discrimination of any kind can cause a lot of stress. Remember the techniques you learned in Chapter 4 to deal with stress so that it does not turn into a health issue or burnout. Include exercise and meditation into your regular routine no matter how busy you are. Eat a healthy, balanced diet. Journal about your feelings and talk with others that you trust.

Chapter Summary and Putting it into Action

Summary
Any type of harassment or discrimination is illegal in your nursing program or workplace, and you have the right to stand up for yourself and demand it to stop.

Dealing with Instructor Problems

Everyone has their share of "tough teachers" during their nursing program. Learning how to deal with them will make you a better nurse.

-        Set up a meeting and ask how you can do better in their class. You will typically learn that they have your best interests at heart.

-        Report them if you are unable to resolve the issue with a face-to-face meeting or you are experiencing a very serious issue like harassment or racial discrimination. Talk to the office of student affairs or whatever the equivalent is at your school and find out the process required to file a complaint.

-        Be confident and kind. Be professional at all times.

Bullying

The American Nurses Association defines bullying as "repeated, unwanted harmful actions intended to humiliate, offend and cause distress in the recipient." Unfortunately, bullying is common in nursing programs and the workplace.

How to Deal with a Bully:

Don't Retaliate: It's not worth it. Retaliating may lead to violence and even getting kicked out of your program.

Examine Yourself: Bullying is never your fault. However, recognizing your part in the situation (if any) may help you start a conversation with this person and come to an understanding that ends the bullying.

Take Advantage of the Resources Available to You: Check with your learning center or school administration offices to see what is available to you.

Stand up to the Bully: Calmly, but firmly state that you will not tolerate this ill-treatment any longer.

Report the Bully: If you are not able to resolve the matter with the bully directly, you have the right to talk to your administrator.

Racial and Gender Discrimination

- "The law forbids discrimination when it comes to any aspect of employment, including hiring, firing, pay, job assignments, promotions, layoff, training, fringe benefits, and any other term or condition of employment."

- If you ever find yourself the victim of discrimination of any kind, you have the legal right to speak up for yourself and expect it to stop.

- Gender bias and discrimination is against the law and should never be considered normal or a small matter.

Tips to Deal with Bullying and Discrimination in the Workplace or School

Don't Wait Too Long to Say Something: The best time to address a bully or discriminator is as soon as you know for sure what is going on. As motivational speaker Lisa Nichols likes to say, "we teach people how to treat us."

Vent, But Don't Gossip: If you need to vent, wait until after hours and talk over the phone or at another location to avoid having someone else overhear your conversation. It's always best to address the offending party first before discussing the matter with others when possible.

Try to Stay Calm: When addressing the situation with the offending party or an administrator, try to stay calm and simply state the facts.

Keep Track of the Details: If you think that you might need to report someone, keep careful notes about the offensive actions with dates, times, locations, etc.

Dominate the Stress: Use the techniques you learned in Chapter 4 to deal with stress so that it does not turn into a health issue or burnout.

Notes

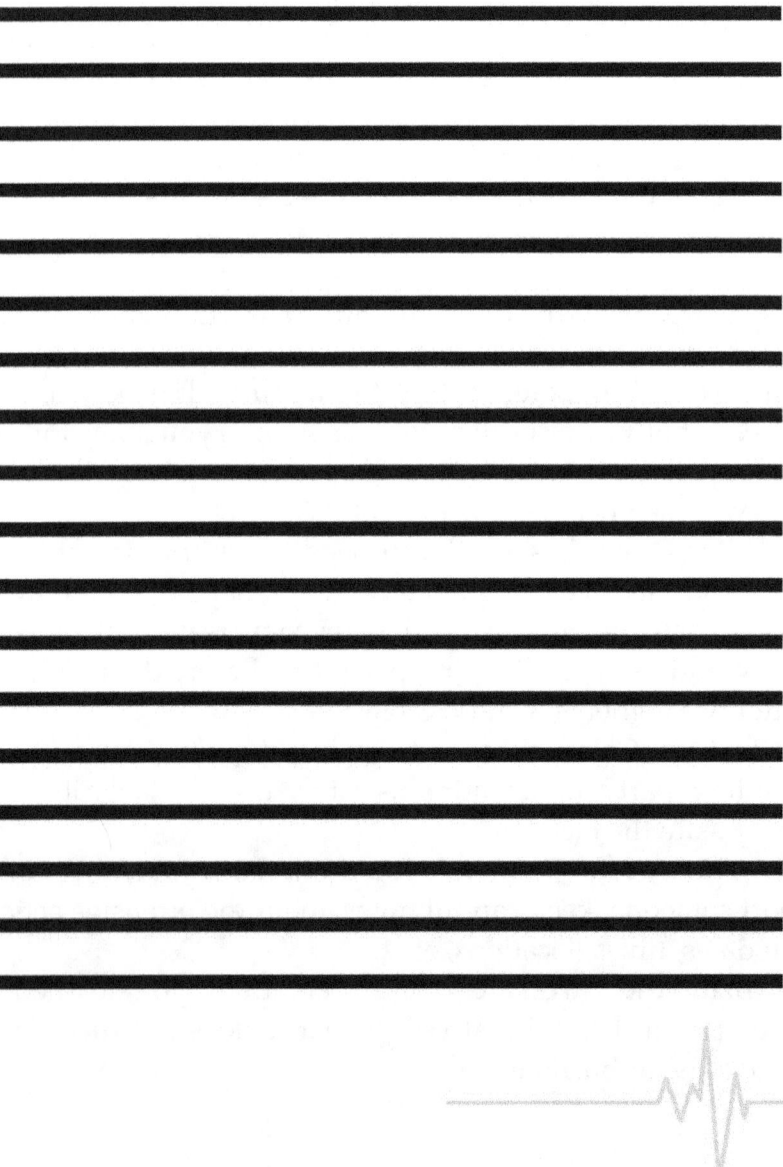

Chapter Nine

Everything You Need to Know About NCLEX

"The trained nurse has become one of the great blessings of humanity, taking a place beside the physician and the priest." William Osler

The NCLEX Breakdown

National Council Licensure Examination (NCLEX) is a nationwide exam to license a nurse in the US or Canada. The purpose of this exam is to test how prepared you are for entry-level nursing work. Over 5 million people have taken the NCLEX over the last twenty-five years, so you will be in good company when you start to prepare for this important step in your nursing career, officially becoming a registered nurse!

How to Register for the NCLEX

About six weeks prior to your graduation, you should receive two applications from your nursing school: an application for a license and an application to take the NCLEX. You can also contact your Nursing Regulatory Body (NRB) to request these applications.

Send in your application and pay your exam fee: You will need to submit both application forms and licensure fees by a specific deadline, so read through the application forms carefully to make sure that you take care of everything in a timely manner.

When your Nursing Regulatory Body decides that you are eligible to take the NCLEX, you will receive an Authorization To Test (ATT) via email. You will need the ATT email to schedule your test, so contact your Nursing Regulatory Body if you don't receive it. Once you receive your ATT, you must schedule your test during the validity period (typically 90 days) and pay a nonrefundable $200 exam fee. This time period cannot be extended for any reason, so make it a priority to get your exam scheduled.

Schedule your exam: Contact Pearson VUE by phone, mail, or online to schedule your exam. Visit www.pearsonvue.com for more information or to register online. Make sure the name you register with matches exactly with the name printed on the identification that you bring with you to the testing center, otherwise you will not be allowed to take your test and you will have to re-register and pay for the exam fee again.

What to Expect on the NCLEX
The NCLEX exams are standardized computer adaptive tests that are made up of mostly multiple choice questions. You will also find drag-and-drop, fill-in-the-blank, and multiple response questions. You may need to answer anywhere between 75 to 265 questions depending on how well you are answering the questions. You have up to 5 hours to complete the NCLEX-PN and up to 6 hours for the NCLEX-RN.

The computer will assess which question you receive by how well you answered the previous question. When you get an answer correct, the next question will be slightly harder. If you miss a question, the next question will be a bit easier. The computer will continue to give you questions until it is at least 95% confident in your ability to pass (or fail) the exam. If you reach the maximum number of questions, the computer will judge whether you pass or fail based on your overall answers.

Bring These Things to the Test:
Before you get to the testing center, make sure that you have the following items with you. If you don't have these items with you, you will be asked to re-register and pay the exam fee again.

• A signed form of ID with a picture: a driver's license, state/province identification, passport, and U.S. military ID are all acceptable.

• Your Authorization to Test (ATT)

• A snack in case you decide to take a break and a bottle of water

Don't Bring
Do not bring any study materials with you to the testing center. You will be able to utilize a calculator on the computer during the test, so don't bother bringing one from home. Earphones can be provided upon request, but you are not allowed to bring your own.

Get There Early and Be Prepared for High Security
Taking the NCLEX is serious business. Get there at least 30 minutes before your scheduled test and be prepared to show your documentation. You will be fingerprinted, and your palm may be scanned before you enter the testing room. You will also have your picture taken. All of your belongings will be placed in a locker outside of the room. Most testing rooms will consist of 10-15 computers around the perimeter of the room separated by dividers. There are cameras and sensors all over the room to ensure that everyone is on their best behavior.

Completing the Exam and Receiving Your Results

The time it takes for you to complete the exam will vary from the other students in your testing center based on how you are answering the questions. You will know that you have completed the exam when your screen reads, "This test is concluded." You may have a few multiple choice questions about your overall impression of the exam, but this does not count towards your grade.

Once you complete your exam, you will typically receive your results within 6 weeks. Some states offer rapid results within 2 business days for a small fee. Talk to your testing center about this option or visit the NCLEX® candidate website for more information.

Both the NCLEX-PN and NCLEX-RN cover the following 8 subject areas:
• Physiological adaptation:
Fluid/electrolyte imbalances, illness management, medical emergencies, pathophysiology, unexpected response to therapies
• Management of care:
Advocacy, client rights, confidentiality, continuity of care, ethical practice, informed consent, information technology, legal responsibilities, performance improvement

• Reduction of Risk Potential:
Changes/abnormalities in vital signs, diagnostic tests, laboratory values, the potential for complications, therapeutic procedures
• Safety and Infection Control:
Accident/injury prevention, emergency response plan, ergonomic principles, hazardous materials, home safety, safe use of equipment, security plan

• Pharmacological and Parenteral Therapies:

Adverse effects, blood products, dosage calculations, expected outcomes, medication administration, pharmacological pain management
• Basic Care and Comfort:
Assistive devices, elimination, mobility/immobility, nutrition and oral hydration, personal hygiene, rest and sleep
• Psychosocial Integrity:
Abuse and neglect, coping mechanisms, crisis intervention, cultural awareness, family dynamics, grief and loss, mental health, stress management, substance abuse

• Health Promotion and Maintenance:
Aging process, developmental stages, disease prevention, health screening, high-risk behaviors, lifestyle choices, self-care

Tips to Prepare for the NCLEX Exam
Many nursing students become extremely nervous when it comes time to take the NCLEX, but with preparation, there is no reason for you to worry about passing your exam. Here are my nine tips on how to prepare to sail through your NCLEX.

#1 — Plan to spend at least 1-2 months studying for the exam. The NCLEX is a big deal, and it is not something that you can cram for over a week or two and expect to pass. You cannot rely on any experience you might have gained as a nurse tech or aide because every hospital does things differently. You'll need to keep it by the book to pass.

#2 — Obtain a test plan. The NCLEX test plan is an outline that was created to help you understand the format and content you will encounter on the exam. Test plans also include sample test questions and tutorials about different types of exam questions. This information is invaluable to help you get prepared to do your best. Don't skip this step! All information and test plans can be found on the NCSBN website.

#3 — Invest in additional resources. There are a number of resources on the market that you can use to prepare for the NCLEX. Visit your school's learning center to see what materials are available to borrow or read onsite. I included a list of recommended study books in the final chapter of this book that you can find online or at your campus bookstore.

#4 — Put together a study plan. Just as you planned your study schedule for nursing school, you should have a specific study schedule to prepare for your NCLEX. Pull out your planner and schedule which days you will study, along with what you plan to study in each session.

#5 — Don't forget your pomodoros. Use the Pomodoro Technique (short 25-minute study sessions with 5-minute breaks) to prepare for your exam. See Chapter 5 for more details on how to use this powerful study method and why it's so effective.

You cannot cram for this test and do well on it. Your best bet is planning study sessions of a reasonable length every day for at least 2 months in advance of the exam.

#6 — Use practice questions. Utilize practice questions and mock exams in your study sessions. Studies show that practice questions help you recall the information better over the long term. Look up the answers to the questions you got wrong and make notes on the areas that you need to study more. Mock exams will give you a good idea of what the test is like, the subject matter you will encounter, and areas that you are weaker in.

#7 — Schedule your test at an optimal time of day for you. You probably already have a good idea about what time of day you are sharpest at. If you are a morning person, and you tend to be more focused and energetic first thing in the morning, schedule a morning test. If the afternoon is when you are at your best, then plan to take your test in the afternoon.

#8 — Eat right, sleep well, and get rest before the test. A big mistake that a lot of students make is to spend every waking hour studying the week before a big test, skipping sleep and meals in order to study more. Your brain needs proper sleep and healthy, well-balanced meals in order to perform at an optimum level (see Chapter 5 to learn more about how sleep and healthy food impact your ability to recall information). If you begin studying for the NCLEX several weeks before your test, you won't need to pull a bunch of all-nighters. Try to go to sleep early the night before your test and eat a healthy meal before you go to the testing center.

#9 — Go into your exam with confidence. When it's time for you to take your exam, remember that you can do this. You have already proven your ability by graduating from nursing school, now is the time to show you have what it takes to become a registered nurse. Believe in yourself!

What to Do if You Fail the First Time

Although the pass rates for the NCLEX are fairly high, many students have had to retake the test in order to successfully become a registered nurse. The good news is, you can retake the test as many times as you need to pass. You will need to pay the exam fee again every time you take the test.

There is typically a waiting period of 45 days before you can take the test again, depending on where you live. Use this time to study based on the subject areas that you were weak on according to your test results. Use lots of practice questions and mock tests to get prepared. There are also online classes that you can take to better prepare for the exam. Try adding some new resources to your arsenal and see if it helps you to do better on your mock exams.

Chapter Summary and Putting it into Action

Summary
National Council Licensure Examination (NCLEX) is a nationwide exam to license a nurse in the US or Canada. The purpose of this exam is to test how prepared you are for entry-level nursing work.

How to Register for the NCLEX
1.   Send in your application to take the test and a $200 exam fee
2.   Receive your Authorization To Test via email
3.   Schedule your exam by contacting Pearson VUE by phone, mail, or online at http://www.pearsonvue.com
What to Expect
•   Standardized computer adaptive test
•   Mostly multiple choice questions with drag-and-drop, fill-in-the-blank, and multiple response questions
•   You may need to answer anywhere between 75 to 265 questions depending on how well you are answering the questions.
•   You have up to 5 hours to complete the NCLEX-PN and up to 6 hours for the NCLEX-RN

Put it into Action
Top Nine Tips to Prepare for the NCLEX
#1 — Plan to spend at least 1-2 months studying for the exam. The NCLEX is a big deal, and it is not something that you can cram for over a week or two and expect to pass.
#2 — Obtain a test plan. The NCLEX test plan is an outline that was created to help you understand the format and content you

will encounter on the exam. All information and test plans can be found on the NCSBN website.

#3 — Invest in additional resources. Visit your school's learning center to see what materials are available to borrow or read onsite.

#4 — Put together a study plan. Pull out your planner and schedule which days you will study along with what you plan to study each session.

#5 — Don't forget your pomodoros. Use the Pomodoro technique (short 25-minute study sessions with 5-minute breaks) to prepare for your exam.

#6 — Use practice questions. Utilize practice questions and mock exams in your study sessions.

#7 — Schedule your test at an optimal time of day for you.

#8 — Eat right, sleep well, and get rest before the test.

#9 — Go into your exam with confidence. Believe in yourself!

Notes

Chapter Ten

A Few More Quick Tips to Enjoy Nursing School

"Every time you smile at someone, it is an action of love, a gift to that person, a beautiful thing." Mother Teresa

At times, nursing school gets a bad rap for being a miserable time in a nurse's life. It doesn't have to be that way. Nursing school can be one of the most enjoyable times of your life with the right attitude and a few good tips from someone who has been there. I've already given you a ton of tips on how to succeed in nursing school. As we near the end of this book, I want to add on a few more quick tips to help you not only succeed but enjoy nursing school.

Tip #1 — Stay Organized to Avoid Stress
The majority of stress and overwhelm comes from lack of preparation and organization. If you have not already read through the first chapter of this book, (I like to skip ahead in my books too) do yourself a favor and read through Chapter 1 and follow the tips to get yourself organized for nursing school. Organized people are more efficient. Efficient people have more time to do things that they enjoy.

Keep your home clean and your school bag organized so that you aren't always looking for supplies 5 minutes before you need to leave for class. Plan your meals so that you aren't struggling to find something healthy to eat at the end of a long day of lectures and clinical hours. It might sound like a lot of work if you are not used to being this organized, but it is absolutely vital to build these organizational habits if you want to enjoy yourself as a busy nursing student and working nurse.

Tip #2 — **Reward Yourself for Small Milestones**
When you are in the middle of a challenging program, it is easy to just go from one exam to another without taking a moment to appreciate all of the smaller achievements. Take some time to celebrate some of your minor wins. When you pass an exam that you worked really hard on, go out to dinner with a friend or loved one. Get yourself a pedicure or go to a movie to reward yourself for finishing your first month of clinicals. Nursing school can feel like a long process; whatever you like to do, enjoy celebrating along the way.

Tip #3 — **Make Time for Fun Weekly**
As I touched on in the scheduling chapter, it is important to schedule something fun for yourself on a regular basis. Focusing solely on school every day of the week and doing nothing else is an easy way to make yourself miserable until you graduate. In addition to celebrating your small milestones, make time on a weekly basis to do something fun that has nothing to do with nursing school.

Take an exercise class that you enjoy. Play a game of pickup basketball with your friends or watch your favorite sports team on TV. Spend one afternoon reading your favorite novel. Plan a weekly movie night with your best friend. Go out with your friends. Choose any activity that you will look forward to and will allow you to take your mind off of school for at least an hour. Trust me, you can take at least one hour each week to unwind, and you will be a better student because of it.

Tip #4 — Eat and Sleep

Regardless of what anyone tells you, there is no excuse not to eat and sleep as a nursing student. Anyone who tells you that you have to live off of junk food and be chronically sleep deprived to survive nursing school is simply not planning properly.

I'm not saying you should never pull an all-nighter because you probably will a few times during your program, but if you are constantly losing sleep to study, you need to plan better or adjust something in your schedule to get more sleep. Being chronically sleep deprived is horrible for your health, concentration, reaction time, and memory. You have got to prioritize sleep if you want to take care of your health and do your best in school.

Take the time to pack healthy meals and snacks so that you are never walking around cranky from hunger. If you need to grab fast food once and a while on a really busy day, that's fine, but you shouldn't make it a habit. Your health and your mood will pay for it.

Happy people eat good food and sleep. Do both!

Tip #5 — **Be Mindful of the Moment**

Sometimes we get so caught up in thinking of all of the demands on our life that we forget to enjoy the task that we are working on at the time. Mindfulness has been a huge movement over the last decade because so many of us are stressed out about achieving goals and making more money. Busyness became a status symbol, until we started seeing a sharp increase in stress-related diseases and mental health problems.

Practice focusing on enjoying the current task that you are working on and forgetting about everything else. When you are studying anatomy, allow yourself to enjoy learning how unique and beautiful the human body is. Forget about the test you have next week, don't worry about your son's basketball game tomorrow night; keep your focus on the task at hand and allow yourself to enjoy it. You'll have plenty of time to focus on everything else after. It's easier said than done, but with practice, you can learn to be mindful of each moment.

Tip #6 — **Think of College as Preparation for Your *Dream Job***
This tip might sound like common sense, but I want you to focus on the words *dream job*. Many students are only focused on passing their program and finding a decent paying job after graduation. As I suggested in earlier chapters, successful students set goals beyond just passing their classes and graduating. Create a vision for yourself of your dream job and keep that vision in front of you throughout your program. If you could work anywhere in the world, where would you work? Would you love to be a traveling nurse and see the world? Do you dream of working with kids or making a difference at a rehab facility? Now is the time to start preparing for your dream job.

Write down your vision and place at it at the front of your notebook or on your bathroom mirror to remind you daily of what you are working so hard for. You might be surprised at the amount of valuable connections and opportunities that will seem to come out of nowhere when you have a clear vision of where you want to go.

Chapter Summary

Quick Tips to Enjoy Nursing School
Tip #1 — Stay organized to avoid stress.
Tip #2 — Reward yourself for small milestones.

Tip #3 — Make time for fun weekly.

Tip #4 — Eat and sleep.

Tip #5 — Be mindful of the moment.

Tip #6 — Think of college as preparation for your dream job.

Notes

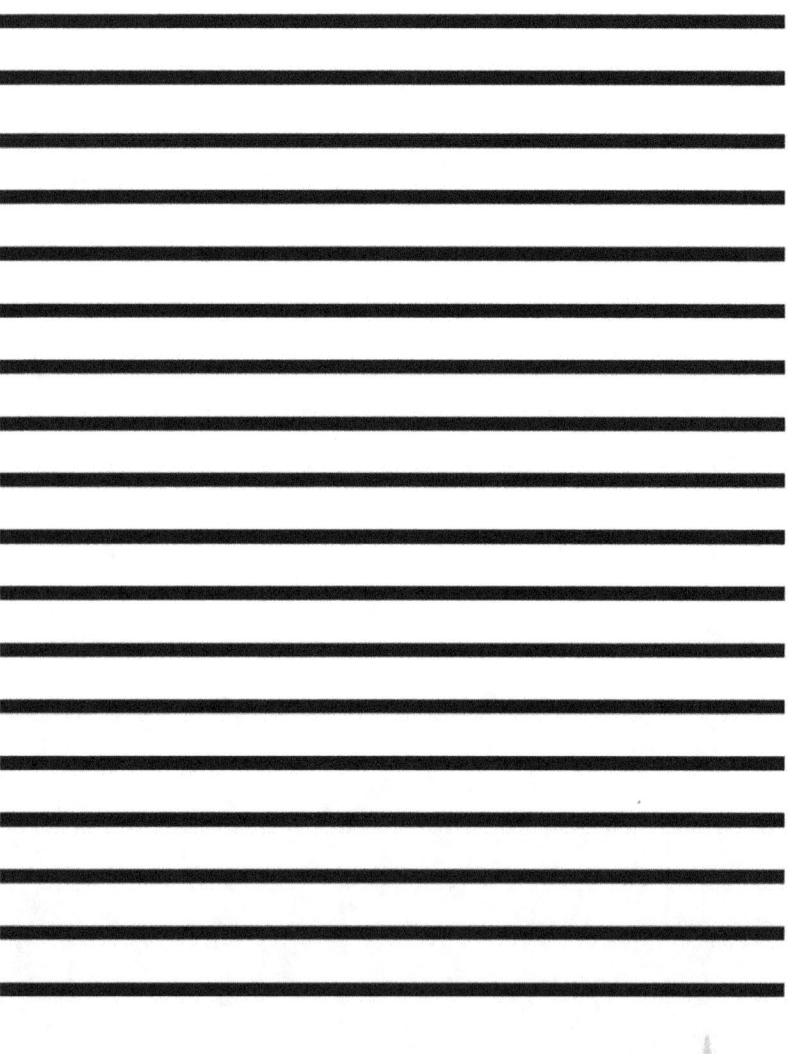

Chapter Eleven

Beyond Nursing School

"I attribute my success to this; I never gave nor took any excuse."
Florence Nightingale

As you are sailing your way through nursing school, it's important to look towards your bright future as a working nurse. I thought it would be helpful to include a few tips in this last chapter to prepare you for life beyond nursing school.

8 Surprising Things About Being a Nurse
1.   Nurses provide MUCH more than medical care on a daily basis. You will be an advocate for your patient, a companion, therapist, housekeeper, waitress, technology expert, and a mediator between your patients, their families, and their doctors.

2.   Nursing school cannot prepare you to deal with witnessing death. Every death you see will affect you in a different way. Unfortunately, there is no way to really prepare yourself for how you are going to react. When you find yourself having a difficult time, talk to a coworker, mentor, or a friend about how you're feeling.

3.   You will make life-long friends at work. Although every workplace has its share of bullies, gossips, and cliques, you are sure to find some life-long friends in your coworkers. No one in your life will understand what you deal with on a daily basis like your coworkers. You'll spend long nights and holidays together. Working together as a team to provide the best care for your patients on a daily basis will bond you together.

4.   You will experience aches in your body that you've never felt before. The fittest athlete might be challenged by taking on a week of 12-plus hour nursing shifts full of bending, lifting patients, standing, and walking with very little breaks. Hopefully, you are taking my advice to exercise regularly and eat a healthy diet to prevent back and joint problems that are common in our industry. Be sure to stay hydrated too. Your body needs plenty of water to function at its best.

5.   Your memory will be tested on a daily basis. Your patients and the doctors you work with will be relying on you to remember important information on disease processes, medications, when medications were given, lab schedules, etc. Write everything down and keep important charts and pocket guides on hand.

6.   Family and friends will text you pictures of every rash and bug bite for the rest of your life. Get ready to hear in-depth health stories from everyone. You will forever be the go-to person in the family for medical advice. It can get a bit annoying at times, but it can be nice to help.

7.   Every nurse makes mistakes. Unfortunately, no amount of preparation will make you mistake-proof. When you do make a mistake, learn from it, and try not to beat yourself up about it. It can be hard to deal with a mistake that negatively affects your patient, but it's important to allow yourself to let it go so that it doesn't shake your confidence. Talk with a mentor

or coworker about how they deal with mistakes. It can be helpful to know that you're not the only nurse that has ever made a mistake.

8.	Nursing is even more rewarding than it seems. There are few professions that allow you to directly impact the lives of others on a daily basis quite like a nurse. It feels wonderful to know that you are saving and enriching the lives of your patients. If you love to learn, you have chosen the right profession because the learning will never stop. You will learn something new every day. You've worked hard to become a working nurse, enjoy it!

Tips to Find Your Dream Nursing Job

Begin with a Clear Vision

If you've followed along with previous chapters and set your goals, you should already have a clear vision of your dream nursing job. If you don't, I strongly suggest taking some time to consider what your dream job will be. While I'm not suggesting that you will be able to land your dream job fresh off of passing your NCLEX, I do think that it's imperative to know where you want to end up.

Having a clear vision for the job that you would like to have will help you make decisions on the jobs you take, the contacts you seek, and the learning opportunities that you pursue on the road to get to where you want to be. Search for your dream job online and print off the job descriptions. Consider how you can work backward from that job to obtain the skills and experience you need to qualify. Don't be afraid to think big and go after what you want.

Obtain References

Before you begin applying for jobs, you should talk to at least five people who can attest to your experience, work ethic, and character. A good reference can sometimes tip the scales in your favor when you are up against another candidate with similar experience and skills, so take this seriously. You should have a good mix of references from instructors and previous employers.

Put Together a Strong Cover Letter and Resume
It goes without saying that a strong cover letter and resume can get your foot in the door. Your resume should showcase your credentials, skills, accomplishments, and relevant experience. The cover letter should focus on why you are a good candidate for the position.

Here are a few tips on how to write a winning cover letter and resume:

Utilize the career center at your school for help. You'd be surprised at how few students utilize the career development resources available to them. Don't make the mistake of trying to figure out everything on your own. Bring your resume into your career center and ask for advice on how to make it better. While you're there, talk to your advisor about your dream job, and ask what you can do to build the experience and skills to get there. You've paid a lot of money to get your education and have access to these resources, use them!

Customize your cover letter and resume for each position that you are applying for. While the base of your resume will stay the same, you want to make it seem that your resume was custom written to fill the job description. Highlight any relevant skills and experience you have that is listed in the job listing. Employers can tell when you are simply sending the same canned cover letter and resume, so simply taking a few extra minutes to customize it will make you stand out.

Use relevant keywords from the job description. Employers will often only look at resumes and cover letters that include specific keywords. Take the time to incorporate as many key phrases as you can for your resume.

Avoid fancy fonts or layouts if you are sending electronically. You never know how this will show up on other computers. Save the fancy layouts for the resumes that you print out to bring to job fairs or interviews.

Have your resume and cover letter proofread before you send it out. No matter how many times you've read over your resume and cover letter, you should always have someone check it for silly typos and grammar mistakes before you send it out. It's very easy to overlook your own mistakes.

Tap into Your Network First
You might be surprised to learn that the majority of jobs do not come from job listings, they come from your network. As you are approaching graduation, you should already begin making as many contacts as you can and letting people know what kind of job you are looking for. You never know who someone may know who can connect you with a job vacancy that is perfect for you. Always be polite and respectful when meeting a potential contact. Ask questions and stay open to potential opportunities.

Utilize Social Media in Your Job Search
Your network also includes your social networks. If you have not already joined a few social media groups for nurses, take a look at the recommended groups in the next chapter and start making contacts. Many of these groups list jobs that aren't always advertised on the job boards, so this can be a wonderful resource for leads.

LinkedIn is perhaps the most powerful social network to connect with potential employers. You can tailor your LinkedIn profile to your job search by making it clear what type of job you are looking for and what your experience is. Recruiters often search this website to find candidates for their clients, so be sure to set your profile settings to specify that you are actively looking for a job and are willing to connect with recruiters. Make sure that you have a clear and professional looking profile picture, and read your entire profile out loud to catch any typos or mistakes. Better yet, ask a friend to proofread your profile for you.

Search for and follow your dream employers and stay up to date on any company news. If you are able to make a personal connection with someone at the company, take the opportunity to express your interest in working with the company, and ask what they look for in potential employees.

Search Job Listings Wisely

It is important to be wise about how much time you spend searching and responding to job listings because only about 3% of jobs are obtained this way. Tap into your network, tap into resources in your career center, and make connections online, then apply to a few select jobs. Search according to your specialty, skills, and experience. Don't waste your time applying to just any nursing job in your area. Your time would be better spent making personal connections through your network.

Build the Experience You Need

You might find it difficult to overcome a lack of experience as a brand-new grad. This is where your school's career center can become an invaluable resource for volunteer and job shadowing opportunities. While it might be hard to think of working for free after you've worked so hard to get your license, some volunteer opportunities will open doors to future jobs that you might not have access to by taking the first job that you can get. You might also be able to find on-call or pier diem work that can lead to full-time work in your specialty. Stay open to any possibility that might lead to your dream job down the line.

Chapter Summary and Putting it into Action

Summary
Eight Surprising Things About Being a Nurse
1.   Nurses provide MUCH more than medical care on a daily basis.
2.   Nursing school cannot prepare you to deal with witnessing death.
3.   You will make lifelong friends at work.
4.   You will experience aches in your body that you've never dealt with before.
5.   Your memory will be tested on a daily basis.
6.   Family and friends will text you pictures of every rash and bug bite for the rest of your life.
7.   Every nurse makes mistakes.
8.   Nursing is even more rewarding than it seems.
Tips to Find Your Dream Job
-       Have a clear vision of your dream job. Print out job descriptions of jobs that you'd love to have.
-       Obtain strong references from your instructors and former employers.
-       Tap into your network. Only 3% of jobs come from job listings, so let your friends, family, and contacts know that you are looking for a job.
Utilize Social Media

-    Search job listings and get job search tips
-    Make connections with potential employers and others in your field
-    Follow companies that you would like to work for and ask what they look for in potential employees
-    Post your resume on LinkedIn and connect with companies you are interested in

Build the Experience You Need
-    Visit your learning center for volunteer and job shadowing opportunities
-    Stay open to temporary and on-call positions in your specialty

Put it into Action

Write a Strong Resume and Cover Letter
-    Utilize the resources at your school's career center.
-    Customize your cover letter and resume for each position that you are applying for.
-    Use relevant keywords from the job description.
-    Avoid fancy fonts or layouts if you are sending electronically.
-    Have your resume and cover letter proofread before you send it out.

Notes

Resources for Your Journey

"Unless we are making progress in our nursing every year, every month, every week, take my word for it we are going back." Florence Nightingale

This chapter is full of the best resources to help you sail through nursing school and beyond. Whether you like to read books, listen to audiobooks or podcasts, watch videos, or connect with other nursing students on social media, you will find something here.

Books and Audiobooks

Here are some of the best books to help you continue learning and stay inspired as a nursing student and working nurse. While I have not read all of these books, I only listed the most highly rated books that you should be able to find easily online or through your local bookstore. Happy reading!

General Nursing Books

Here is a mix of the top nonfiction, biographies, and a few novels mixed in for fun. Check online or your local library for audiobook versions for many of these books.

How to Survive and Maybe Even Love Your Life as a Nurse by Keli S. Dunham and Staci J. Smith

Your First Year as a Nurse, Making the Transition from Total Novice to Successful Professional by Donna Cardillo RN

First Year Nurse: Wisdom, Warnings, and What I Wish I'd Known My First 100 Days on the Job (Kaplan Test Prep) by Barbara Arnoldussen

I Wasn't Strong Like This When I Started Out: True Stories of Becoming a Nurse by Lee Gutkind

Nursing Diagnosis Handbook: A Guide to Planning Care by Elizabeth Ackley and Gail Ladwig

Taber's Cyclopedic Medical Dictionary edited by Donald Venes, Clayton L. Thomase, and Clarence Wilbur Taber

The Nurse's Communication Advantage by Kathleen Pagana

Leave No Nurse Behind: Nurses Working with disAbilities by Donna Maheady

Health Assessment & Physical Examination by Mary Ellen Zator Estes

Nursing School Cheat Sheets: 50 Tips for Making the Grade by Donovan Gow

Nursing Mnemonics: 108 Memory Tricks to Demolish Nursing School by Jon Haws

Nursing Ethics in Everyday Practice by Connie M. Ulrich

Inspired Nurse by Rich Bluni, RN

Cooked: An Inner City Nursing Memoir by Carol Karels

Bedham Among the Bedpans: Humor in Nursing by Amy Y. Young

Notes on Nursing: What It Is, and What It Is Not by Florence Nightingale

Dosage Calculations for Nursing Students: Master Dosage Calculations in 24 Hours the Safe and Easy Way Without Formulas by Bradley J. Wojcik and Chase Hassen

When Nurses Hurt Nurses: Recognizing and Overcoming the Cycle of Bullying by Cheryl Dellasega

Ross and Wilson Anatomy and Physiology in Health and Illness by Anne Waugh
Nursing Care Plans: Diagnoses, Interventions, and Outcomes by Meg Gulanick and Judith L. Meyers

The Everything New Nurse Book by Kathy Quan

Rnotes: Nurse's Clinical Pocket Guide by Ehren Myers

Critical Thinking, Clinical Reasoning, and Clinical Judgement in Nursing: A Practical Approach by Rosalinda Alfaro-Lefevre

Helping Children Overcome Fear in a Medical Setting by Rob Luka

Woman of Valor: Clara Barton and the Civil War by Stephen B. Oates

The Immortal Life of Henrietta Lacks by Rebecca Skloot

Exam Preparation
Make sure that you get the latest edition of any of the following books to help you prepare for exams. Your school's learning center may have some of these titles available for you to borrow or read onsite.
ATI TEAS Secret Study Guide: Complete study manual, full-length practice tests, and video tutorials

Saunders Strategies for Test Success: Passing Nursing School and the NCLEX Exam by Linda Anne Silvestri Ph.D. RN and Angela Silvestri MSN RN

Test Success: Test-Taking Techniques for Beginning Nursing Students (Davis's Q&A Success) by Patricia M. Nugent RN MA MS EdD and Barbara A. Vitale RN MA

NCLEX: Fundamentals of Nursing by Chase Hassen

Nursing School Entrance Exams Prep 2019-2020: Your All-In-One Guide to the Kaplan and HESI Exams by Kaplan Nursing

Nursing School Entrance Exams: General Review for the TEAS, HESI, PAX-RN, Kaplan, and PSB-RN Exams by Kaplan Nursing

Review Guide for RN Pre-Entrance Exam by Null

HESI Comprehensive Review for the NCLEX-RN Examination

Evolve Reach: Comprehensive Review for the NCLEX-RN Examination

Lippincott Q&A Review for NCLEX-RN

NCLEX-RN Practice Questions Exam Cram

Prioritization, Delegation, and Assignment: Practice Exercises for the NCLEX Exam

Study Skills and Learning Styles
If you want to dive deeper into how to use your learning style(s) effectively or how to study better in general, here are some resources that will help you.

A Mind for Numbers by Dr. Barbara Oakley will show you how your brain works and how to use this information to learn any topic more effectively (not just numbers as the title suggests).

Spark: The Revolutionary New Science of Exercise and the Brain by John J. Ratey, MD shares some of the latest groundbreaking science to prove how exercise and good nutrition play a vital role in your cognitive function.

Test Success: Test-taking Techniques for Beginning Nursing Students by Patricia M. Nugent RN MA MS EdD and Barbara A. Vitale RN MA includes a complete review of core concepts and over 800 questions to use for study.

Unlimited Memory: How to Use Advanced Learning Strategies to Learn Faster, Remember More, and Be More Productive by Kevin Horsely is a best-selling book on Amazon that will show you useful tips to recall information easily and effectively.

Vital Skills by Kathleen Straker and Eugenia Kelman teaches important study skills that "every nurse must know."

Incredibly Easy Series: If you are a visual learner, you'll want to take a good look at this series of study materials to help you master things like nursing care planning, cardiovascular care, ER care, ECG interpretation, and more.

Nursing Specialties
A Daybook for Critical Care Nurses by Eileen Gallen Bademan

Something for the Pain: Compassion and Burnout in the ER by Paul Austin

Call the Midwife: A Memoir of Birth, Joy, and Hard Times by Jennifer Worth

Wong's Essentials of Pediatric Nursing by Marilyn J. Hockenberry and David Wilson

A Healing Touch: True Stories of Life, Death, and Hospice edited by Richard Russo

Merenstein & Gardner's Handbook of Neonatal Intensive Care by Sandra Lee Gardner, Brian Carter, Mary I Enzman-Hines, and Jacinto Hernandez

The Comfort Garden, Tales from the Trauma Unit by Laurie Barkin

Cardiac Surgery Essentials for Critical Care Nursing by Sonya R. Hardin

Apps for Your Smartphone or Tablet
These apps are designed to help you be more efficient during your clinicals and as a working nurse. You can also use them to study on the go. Most of these apps are available for both IOS and Android. Search your favorite app store to download the apps that interest you. I tried to include a good mix of free and paid apps for you to choose from. Please note the prices and descriptions may change, so read the descriptions carefully.

Critical Care ACLS Guide: ($7.99) Convenient guide with rich illustrations to help you read EKGs, avoid drug interactions, and administer correct dosages.

Epocrates Rx: (Free) Helpful pharmacology app for dosing information, contraindications, and administration directions.

Epocrates Essentials: (Paid) Although it's expensive ($159.99), it provides access to a full encyclopedia of drug information, anatomy, symptom, and disease guides, as well as a rundown of other helpful apps.

Eponyms (for students): (Free) Use this app to quickly look up the meaning of any eponyms.

Heart Murmur Pro: ($3.99) Listen and understand heart sounds with over 23 sounds available and access to medical databases.

OB Wheel: ($1.99) Digital version of the paper wheel that you are used to but allows for more flexibility due to irregularities and you can have it on hand at all times.

Pill Identifier: (.99) Search over 10,000 pills by shape, color, strength, and more.

Med Mnemonics: ($1.99) Handy app for both nursing students and working nurses.

Medscape: (Free) Many hospitals offer Medscape as a resource in their intranet. It is useful to find answers to any random question you might have during a shift and read the latest medical news.

Medical Spanish by Marvo: (Free) Very helpful app if you don't speak Spanish. It includes audio and commonly used phrases in a medical setting to help you communicate with your patients and provide the best care.

NCSBN Learning Extensions Medication Flashcards: (Free) This convenient app includes a full medication library that you can use on the go.

NurseGrid: (Free) A convenient scheduling app made by nurses and for nurses and nursing students. It's useful to plan study sessions with classmates and share your schedule.

PediSTAT: ($4.99) Must-have app for nurses in emergency or pediatric care. Use it to calculate medication for children, analyze symptoms, and get descriptions of procedures.

Pocket Lab Values: ($2.99) Access over 320 common and uncommon lab values right on your phone.

Pocket Body: Musculoskeletal: ($2.99) Comprehensive guide of the musculoskeletal system created by Pocket Academy is helpful to refresh your memory after graduation or use it to study during nursing school

Scrubcheats: (Free, but you will need to purchase the cheat packs) Scrub cheats created by NRSNG are extremely popular study aids that you can carry around with you to remember important information. The app includes all of the same information with the convenience of full access on your smartphone or tablet.

Skyscape Medical Resources: (Free) Useful app that includes a medical calculator, drug information, medical news, and a database of medical journals.

Symptomia: (Free) Allows you to look up symptoms, possible causes, and diagnosis quickly.

Taber's Medical Dictionary: ($39.99) Use this app to find the definition of any medical term that you don't understand. It includes over 1200 photo illustrations and 100 videos.

WebMD: (Free) Although patients might use this app to incorrectly self-diagnose, it can be useful for symptom, disease, and other medical questions you might have during clinicals.

Blogs and Websites to Follow

General Nursing Blogs and Websites
American Nurses Association (nursingworld.org) is the website to follow for all aspiring nurses. Read about nursing practice and policy as well as the latest news in our field.

DailyNurse (dailynurse.com) "The Pulse of Nursing" gives you up-to-date advice, job listings, and scholarship information for nursing programs.

FreshRN (freshrn.com) offers a helpful blog with NCLEX study strategies, new nurse survival tips, product reviews, how to deal with burnout, and more. This website also offers helpful courses, books, and gear.

Minority Nurse (minoritynurse.com): Minority Nurse magazine created a blog to inform under-represented populations in nursing. They offer scholarship information, job listings, and the latest news.

NRSNG (nrsng.com): This popular website provides a wealth of advice, courses, videos, and resources to help you effectively study for exams and become the best nurse that you can be.

Nurse.org (nurse.org): Learn more about nursing programs, read hospital reviews, search for jobs, and more.

Nurse Buff (nursebuff.com): Humor and lifestyle blog for nurses that includes memes to entertain you, mnemonics that you won't forget, and more.

Nurse Code (nursecode.com): Nurse Beth started her blog to help nurses land the right job for them and excel in their careers.

Nurse Journal (nursejournal.org) is a social community for nurses worldwide that provides information on entry-level nursing, nursing degrees, and advanced studies.

Simple Nursing (simplenursing.com) is a subscription website containing over 1,200 videos and 200 study guides to help you study for nursing exams and understand important concepts.

Nursing Jobs
The following websites will help you find nursing job listings in your area.

Indeed (indeed.com) — General job search website that includes nursing jobs nationwide

Monster (monster.com) — General job search website that includes nursing jobs nationwide

Nurse.com — Jobs and continuing education courses

NursingJobs (nursingjobs.com) — Lists permanent, per diem, and travel nursing jobs

NursingJobCafe (nursingjobcafe.com) — Offers thousands of active jobs in various specialties

Podcasts
Podcasts are an easy way to learn on the go. Subscribe to your favorite podcasts to learn while you exercise, drive, or cook dinner. Listening to a podcast before going to bed can be a good replacement for watching TV because the blue light from television sets and phones can disrupt your sleep cycles and make it harder to fall asleep. Some studies suggest that studying right before bed may even improve memory and recall.

The Nursing Show by Jamie Davis: Jamie Davis' podcast offers weekly news, interviews, tips, and medical information for nurses.

Medical Spanish Podcasts by Molly Martin, MD: Listen to Spanish conversations in common medical encounters to brush up on your Spanish vocabulary and grammar with this app.

Nursing Podcast by NRSNG: Nurse Jon Hawes created this helpful and inspiring podcast for nursing students to learn how to study for exams and succeed in nursing school.

Nursing Uncensored: This is a podcast full of real conversations about the life of a nurse.

Real Talk School of Nursing: This podcast was started by two nursing students to share their experiences and help other students through nursing school.

Ted Talks Health: Highly popular Ted Talks Health offers short digestible episodes to keep you informed about important health and medical information.

Trauma Nursing to Go: This is an educational podcast for trauma nurses.

The Nurse Keith Show by Keith Carlson, RN, BSN, NC-BC: Nurse Keith offers career advice for the 21st century nurse.

YouTube channels
Online videos are a fun way to learn about almost any topic under the sun. Check out the following YouTube channels created specifically for nurses and nursing students. You can simply type the title of the channel in the YouTube search bar to access it. If you subscribe to the channel, you will be notified about new videos so you don't miss any.

Future Nurse Abby: Watch Abby's journey through nursing school and learn from her mistakes and successes.

Nurse Bass: Nurse Bass includes helpful tips for nursing students and practicing nurses.

Nurse Liz: Adventures of a Nurse Practitioner: This channel offers some valuable videos for how to survive nursing school and what to expect after graduation.

The Nurse Nook with Alexis Nicole, RN: Alexis includes videos about her nursing school journey and her life as an RN.

Registered Nurse RN: This channel has videos on how to study for the NCLEX, lectures on various specialties, and job interview tips.

Facebook Groups

Social media groups and forums are an easy way to find a community that understands the unique journey that you are on as a nursing student or working nurse. To find any of the following groups, simply type in the title of the group into the search bar under the Facebook groups tab. If a group is labeled as "closed," you may need to request an invitation to join the group by contacting the group's administrator.

You can find hundreds of more groups by searching "nurses" or "<your specialty> nursing" under the groups tab on Facebook.

AllNursingStudents: Find other nursing students around the world to share your journey with.

American Nurses Association: Like the ANA website, this is a must-follow social channel for nursing students and registered nurses for news in your industry, tools to find your first job, and more.

Nurse Health Project: This group is for nurses who are dealing with burnout, stress, or job-related health issues.

NSNA Inc.: This group is specifically for nursing students.

Nursing Life: General Facebook page for nurses to connect.

Nursing Link: This page by Monster.com focuses on job leads and tips for nurses.

Black Nurses Rock: This group brings nurses together worldwide with stories and discussions.

Nurse Rounds: Nurse Rounds is a general Facebook page for nurses to connect.

Nurse Together: Join this community for nursing and lifestyle advice.

Nurse Up: Nurse Up is focused on nursing entrepreneurship.

Student Nurses: This is a place to vent your frustrations, ask questions, and share your journey as a student.

The Travel Nurse (The Gypsy Nurse): Over 10,000 members enjoy following Nurse Candy as she travels around the world.

Miscellaneous Nursing Supplies
As you are shopping for your essential nursing supplies (see Chapter 1 for my suggested shopping list), take a look at the following companies.

All Heart (www.allheart.com)
All Heart calls itself America's Medical Superstore. You can find deals on everything from lab coats to stethoscopes. Look out for free shipping codes for this website.

Couture Scrubs and Fashion
(www.couturescrubsandfashion.com)
I am very proud to introduce you to my company. Couture Scrubs and Fashion is an online boutique with the latest fashion must-haves. Find easy fits for various body types, great customer service, and amazing prices.

Hopkins Medical Supplies
(www.hopkinsmedicalproducts.com)
Hopkins Medical Supplies has been around since 1945 and offers a large selection of nursing supplies. Free shipping is available.

Medical Equipment Affiliates (www.meaok.com)
This website offers a wide variety of customized equipment kits for every specialty and a large selection of instruments.

Nurse Mates (www.nursemates.com)
Nurse Mates sells a wide variety of scrubs, nursing shoes, compression socks, nursing bags, and more.

About the Author

Wynisha Alcorn MSN, RN is a fully licensed and Registered Nurse who has a Master's in Nursing. Having worked for 15 years, she practically has an adequate amount of experiences in all levels of nursing. At both staff and management levels, she has worked in environments where the stress was high and the pay was low, and vice versa. She understands the proven traits that makes nurses successful are being a great communicator, understanding that the level of respect received will always be a reflection of what is given, but still remain diplomatic and express empathy for the pain and suffering of others. These traits, along with a heavy dose of enthusiasm encouraged(strong-armed) her, assisting in the decision to provide aspiring medical professionals with proven recipes through various tools. She is also a Certified Life Professional Coach (CPLC). While in nursing school, Wynisha underwent a lot of "tribulations" as a mother and as a Nurse, and that gave her the motivating force to provide support to other students out there in nursing schools, clinicals, labs, and so on.

Other Resources by Wynisha Alcorn MSN, RN

Couture Scrubs and Fashion
www.couturescrubsandfashion.com
Couture Scrubs and Fashion is an online boutique with the latest fashion must-haves. Find easy fits for various body types, great customer service, and amazing prices.

Dating2Love App is now available on Google Play at
https://www.dating2love.com/

Dating2Love is an app for single people to meet face-to-face with likeminded people and spark conversations with the potential for romance. If you are looking for that special someone or just fancy a fun night out meeting new people, Dating2Love is waiting for you!

www.ingramcontent.com/pod-product-compliance
Lightning Source LLC
Chambersburg PA
CBHW060851170526
45158CB00001B/310